Worst Diet Ever

how to find the motivation to lose weight and live healthy

2nd Edition

Including what employers, insurance companies, and governments can do to keep their employees, customers, and citizens healthy

By Yoram Solomon, PhD

Yoram Solomon © 2014-2017

*For those who put their lives on the line to
protect our freedom.*

Worst Diet Ever

2nd Edition

How to find the motivation to lose weight and live healthy

TABLE OF CONTENTS

"God grant me the serenity
to accept the things I cannot change;
courage to change the things I can;
and wisdom to know the difference.
Living one day at a time;
enjoying one moment at a time;
accepting hardships as the pathway to peace."

(from the Serenity Prayer by Robert NieBuhr)

INTRODUCTION

Every summer my wife and two daughters, Maya and Shira, fly to Israel for three to four weeks to visit the family. As my parents are long gone, and as much as I do get along well with my in-laws, I don't typically join them. It's a long flight, and it's pretty hard for me to get away from my work and my community involvement for such a long time. Not to mention that I have the opportunity to build my airplanes in every room of the house for three weeks. However, we typically combine their trip to Israel with a family trip in the US or Europe. Here is how we do it: they fly to Israel, and on their way back, because American Airlines has never been able to connect them back to Dallas on the same day, we extend their overnight stay and turn it into a five or so days stay in their connecting airport. I then fly to meet them at that airport, rent a car, and we travel for a week or so. In 2012 they stayed in New York for five days. I joined them, and we planned a five day packed trip to Washington D.C. and New York City. We visited museums, government offices, the World Trade Center, and many other attractions, including the Hershey chocolate factory (not a great place to start a diet).

On the last day, given that our flight back to Dallas was not until the evening, we decided to leave our luggage at the hotel and took the subway to the Rockefeller Plaza. I should add that our main TV network at home is NBC, and we watch the early part of The TODAY Show every morning. So that morning we headed there. We stood by the fence and jumped and waved when the anchors came out. After a while, we decided to go into their "experience store" on the second floor of the GE building. This was at the time of the 2012 London Olympics, and the store had plenty of memorabilia and accessories associated with it. As I was browsing through different shirts, three people approached me. One was wearing makeup for "on air" performance (I did not recognize her at the time, but she was NBC's nutrition editor Madelyn Ferstrom), and the other two carried clipboards.

"Would you like to appear on The TODAY Show this morning?" one of them asked. I looked down at my watch, and realized it was already past 9am.

"Isn't the TODAY show over by now?" I replied with a question. Maya, who overheard the conversation, immediately jumped and stood by my side with keen interest.

"Oh, we're talking about the later part of The TODAY Show, that started at 9am. The part with Kathie Lee Gifford and Hoda Kotb".

"What do you want me on the show for?" I further asked.

"It's about weight loss," they carefully answered. I looked down to see what was it that made them seek me out for a show about weight loss. But, hey, any reason is a good reason to be on TV, right? And this was not just *any* TV show, it was The TODAY show!

"What do you need me to do?"

"Every morning we turn to the audience to see if there are any questions. We need you to ask a question associated with weight loss. If you have a question we like, we would like you to ask it on air".

I thought for a second and realized I actually had a good question—very good question.

"OK, how's this: I know what I have to do to lose weight. I know how I need to eat, and I know how I need to exercise. I know what I should and shouldn't do, but where do you get the motivation?"

"Oh, this is a great question! Let's put him on air," said Madelyn Ferstrom. The others immediately took notes on their clipboards, and then invited me to another room, where I would get some makeup myself. After all, we don't want me to shine on TV too much.

"Can I ask a question, too?" asked Maya.

"Well, dear, what is your question?" They asked her gently.

"How can we, the rest of the family, help him lose weight?" Actually, not a bad question at all. And after all, Maya wanted to be on TV as well. Shira didn't care as much.

"That's a good question too! Why don't you come with your dad to the show?" Maya was thrilled.

We went to the preparation room and then to a room where many others who were invited to ask questions on the show were standing. I guess we weren't the only ones. However, they did put us in the front row, and we got to ask the first question. So I asked the question I had. The answer was pretty generic: "You need to take small steps. Those will motivate you. And you also need to get the support of others." (There went Maya's question that she never got to ask on air). And that was it[1]. After we got the answer we left that room, finished our shopping at the NBC experience store, collected our luggage from the hotel, and flew back to Dallas.

But what happened next led to the writing of this book.

***

I was a skinny child. But for a while now I've been struggling with losing weight. I don't think I was ever obese, although I was borderline. I was definitely overweight. I don't believe there is an absolute right chart for how much should I weigh, but I'm pretty sure I weighed too much. WebMD has a nice calculator[2] to calculate your Body Mass Index (BMI) and your healthy weight range. It claims that my healthy weight should be between 140 and 189 pounds (but my current physician doesn't want me to be under 200). At every physical exam my physician would tell me that I needed to lose weight. I needed to exercise more (which, compared to not exercising at all, anything would be *more*), and I needed to cut down carbs, or fats, or what have you. Every few years I switched to a new doctor, but they all seemed to want the same things, so that didn't help.

And then, in my annual physical examination in January of 2012, I had a blood test done that was much more comprehensive. It was sent to the Boston Heart Diagnostics center[3]. Not only that it

---

[1] http://video.today.msnbc.msn.com/today/48210533#48210533
[2] http://www.webmd.com/diet/calc-bmi-plus
[3] http://www.bostonheartdiagnostics.com/index.php

                                    Yoram Solomon

measured my cholesterol level, but it also measured the amount of large and small, good and bad cholesterol molecules[4]. With this test, you get six monthly consultations with a nutritionist. Free. This was probably the most comprehensive nutritional education I had ever received. The sessions even included a trip to a local "Market Street" to read food labels and learn how to make the right choices. I certainly learned a lot. I'm not being cynical or sarcastic. The session always started with a weigh-in. And then we talked. She taught me about nutrition, and I told her about the products I'm developing, my hobbies, and everything else I could talk about. She would ask me if I paid attention to what I ate, and the answer will typically be *no.* Then, at the beginning of the last session, we measured my weight for the last time. But then, I asked her to check what my weight was when we first started. She looked up the numbers on her computer screen, and then her face turned red. I *gained* eighteen pounds during the six months I was educated by her. Now, this was not her fault. She taught me what I *needed* to do. I knew what I needed to do. I just didn't do it. This was probably when I realized that knowledge is not the issue. The real issue was motivation. I didn't have any, and I didn't know why. Less than two weeks later I was to ask this question on national TV.

***

So you just bought another book about weight loss. Or this was your first one? (In which case—I'm honored!) Why do we buy all those books about weight loss? Why do we spend hundreds and thousands of dollars on weight loss products and programs? Market

---

4 http://www.bostonheartdiagnostics.com/science_portfolio_map_test.php

Data Enterprises published a report[5] that claimed that the US market for weight loss products and services was 60.5 billion dollars in 2013! This means that on average every American (including newborn babies) spent almost 200 dollars on weight loss that year. Every American. You spent $10 just now.

So why do we do it? Because dieting is hard, and we are lazy. The positive consequences of a good diet are so far into the future, yet the temptations are so immediate. We like to eat. Food makes us happy. Desserts and sweets make are even happier. We don't like to exercise. Exercise makes us sad. So we are looking for the silver bullet: maybe a book that would teach us what to eat so that we will feel full and happy, yet not gain weight; maybe some electronic device with electrodes that will exercise our muscles such that we will lose weight while we're asleep. And why? Because we have very little motivation, so we lose weight only if it is easy.

But there is no silver bullet. Dieting is hard. And in order to do something hard for the rest of your life, you need to have strong motivation. So this book is not about an *easy* diet that fits our little to no motivation, because it doesn't exist. This book is about creating *strong* motivation to go through a hard diet and to stay healthy for the rest of your life.

***

As I started writing this book, I realized that, as part of it, I needed to develop a survey to support (or reject) my hypotheses made through it. Between April 15 and April 23 of 2014 I conducted

---

[5] http://www.prweb.com/releases/2014/02/prweb11554790.htm

                                          Yoram Solomon

the survey. It was a short, 10-question survey that took less than one minute to complete. It took eight days to gather more than 200 responses, and I closed with 222 responses in total.

Throughout this book I will highlight results from this survey, but, for now, I will only say that it strongly supported what this book is about to tell you. Did I follow the exact guidelines for doctorate level research? Not really. Close to it. Close enough. I will also not use terms such as "statistical significance" and others that will not make sense to everyone. But I will show you how this all makes sense to *you*.

At this point, let me just share a few high level statistics resulting from the survey. First of all, the survey showed that 86% wanted, needed, or were told they needed to lose weight in the past five years. Of that number, 67% actually lost at least 10 pounds, but only 37% kept at least half of the weight they lost off, 26% of them kept it off for more than 3 months, and only 14% (31 of the original 222 participants) kept more than half of the weight they lost off for more than a year. No doubt, losing weight and keeping the weight you lost off is hard. This helps explain the 60.5 billion dollars spent a year on weight loss products and services. It is interesting to note that of all respondents, more than half (57%) lost less than 10 pounds and only 43% lost more. Less than a quarter of the participants (24%) lost more than 25 pounds, which I would consider a significant loss in weight. There were three major independent variables (or causes) that I measured with this survey: the *frequency* in which a participant measured his or her weight, the *source* of motivation to lose weight (and keep it off), and the *length of time* in which that weight was lost. There were two dependent variables (effects, or results) measured: how much weight was lost and whether the participant was able to keep that weight off long after weight loss occurred. Throughout the book I will analyze the impact of different decisions and choices used by participants on the amount of weight loss and the ability to keep it off over an extended period of time. If interested in the study, more detail about the survey can be found in the last chapter of this book.

***

When it was time for me to choose a methodology for my Ph.D. study on motivation for creativity, I chose qualitative research over quantitative. Although, I did take both quantitative (statistical-explanatory) classes and qualitative (interview-exploratory) classes and did use some statistical analysis in that research, and I am using some here in this book—I like the exploratory nature of the face-to-face interviews. I can hear something that all of a sudden triggers a new line of questions I hadn't thought of before.

This book was no different, and thus I conducted several face-to-face interviews. I learned from each one of them. If it hadn't been for Alex, I wouldn't have thought about the fact that the effort gets lower as it becomes habit. If it hadn't been for Valerie, I wouldn't have thought of the importance of the example you give your child. Without Matthew I wouldn't have thought about the phrase "give the keys to someone else." Don showed me how weight loss was a long-term effort that could become a habit, while both Joe and Alex demonstrated the power of a life-altering statement. Their stories, as they each relate to weight loss, are included here.

***

                    Yoram Solomon

I could wait ten years before publishing this book in an effort to show that I kept my weight off for a long time using the techniques described in this book. I could seek endorsements and reviews from nutrition and diet experts who may, or may not, agree with what I have written here. I could run a seven year clinical trial with two hundred participants to show the efficacy of my method. But I felt a sense of urgency to share this with you *now*.

This book poured out of me. I started writing this book on April 4, 2014. It took me 17 weeks to complete from the moment I typed the first word. By July 31, the book was done. I used Google docs so I could maintain access to the manuscript from wherever I was and on whichever device was convenient. I wrote pieces as emails sent to myself. I even wrote parts of this text on my iPhone, sometimes while working out on the treadmill. This book includes insights I have gathered from different disciplines: psychology, economics, management, and engineering. But more than any of these, I included knowledge gained through common sense and personal experience. Here is my promise: this book will make sense for *you*.

So I'm not making any weight loss promises, which is one of the reasons I haven't called this book "the *best* diet ever." If I did, I would have to prove them, and I didn't want to.

***

There are other reasons why I called the book *The Worst Diet Ever*. Skip this part if you are not interested in knowing why you picked this book over others.

A day after I started writing this book, I was already looking for a name. Something else you need to know: at this point in time, I wanted a Jeep Wrangler Unlimited (the long, four door version). So while on the treadmill, I started looking up YouTube videos and used the search term "Jeep Wrangler Unlimited." A few videos came up. One of them was titled: "Jeep Wrangler Unlimited: The Worst Daily Ride Ever[6]." (It's funny, even when I type these words; this is still the first video that comes up in this search). I immediately watched it.

Why would my car (to be) of choice be the worst ride ever? The narrator claimed that the steering wheel is not telescopic, so it can be a bit hard to reach for short people. I'm tall, so that's not a problem. He said that the engine is noisy, and the ride is rough. Aren't those the reasons why you want to buy a Jeep? I ended up being more convinced than ever that I wanted a Jeep. And then I got it. It was brilliant! I watched this video first because of the negative name! I now knew what I had to do, and I had a name for this book.

If you want to know why this worked, you would have to go to the work of Daniel Kahneman and Amos Tversky, who developed the Prospect Theory[7] in 1979 and won the Nobel Prize in economics in 2002, although Kahneman reportedly never took a single class in economics—he is a Eugene Higgins Professor of Psychology in Princeton University. The Prospect Theory claims that we are much more sensitive to *negative* things (specifically risk and loss) than we are to positive things. The authors claim that "losses hurt more than gains feel good." Recent advances in functional magnetic resonance imaging (MRI), and tests conducted using MRI have demonstrated

---

[6] https://www.youtube.com/watch?v=BS4ERDPr4Vw

[7] http://www.princeton.edu/~kahneman/docs/Publications/prospect_theory.pdf

that decisions are dominated by emotions surrounding *unpredicta-
ble* phenomenon (in this case, the title "worst diet ever"), supporting
Prospect Theory. But I digress. Let's talk about losing weight.

***

To make a long story short (although right after this I will
make the short story long again), I weighed over 230 pounds that
July day in New York. Six months later, and three days ahead of
schedule, on December 29, 2012, my weight was just *under* 200
pounds—199.3 pounds, to be precise. As I was writing these lines, in
April 2014, my weight was still 200 pounds. I didn't gain the weight I
lost back. The purpose of this book is for me to share with you how I
did it and how you can do it yourself.

Many diet techniques were created by passionate people who
lost much more than I have. People who lost even more than 100
pounds used those techniques. I tried few of them, but I didn't try
everything. Somehow, other techniques never worked for me. It
seems they never worked for you, either. Otherwise, why would you
spend more money and time reading *this* book when there are so
many other things you could do? I am not passionate about one single method for losing weight over any other. There are plenty of
books, videos, websites, and other resources out there that can be
used. In fact, I didn't use one method exclusively over others for my
own weight loss because they are all merely tools to reach a goal, and
I focused on the goal. This book is different than any other book on
weight loss. This book is about finding the *motivation* to lose weight.
Once you have the motivation, you will find the tool (or set of tools)
right for *you* that will help achieve *your* goal. My purpose in writing
this book was not even to motivate you *myself,* but rather to teach

you how to find your *own* motivation and harness it to lose weight and to keep that weight off. What motivates you is different than what motivates me.

***

In 2017, I met a Japanese gentleman by the name of Hidetaka Kai. He was visiting Dallas, and was interested in the book and its premise. After some discussion he brought up the fact that in Japan companies (and even the government) are actively participating in helping their employees (and citizens) become healthier. One of the reasons is financial. The cost of unhealthy habits is tremendous. He wanted to know how companies, insurance companies, and the government can use the framework of this book to motivate their employees to be healthy. After an hour-long discussion and whiteboard writing, I modified the framework to address this need. As a result, I added a chapter to this book, and published this second edition.

***

Before you begin reading, a word about my style. I use personal stories throughout this book. They will help you understand things in first person. I am not detached from what I'm telling you. Second, there will be times you will find me cynical and even sarcastic. That's just my sense of humor. I'm working on it.

Yoram Solomon

1.

THE ECONOMICS OF WEIGHT LOSS

This chapter begins describing the core of my theory for weight loss. But before I can explain that, I need to start with three concepts, none of which have anything to do with health, diet, or weight loss. However, the feedback I received from readers of the first edition was that this part might be too complicated. I tried to simplify it, but if you are not up to learning what Net Present Value is—just skip it.

***

The first concept is taken from the field of economics and finance and is called "Net Present Value" (or NPV). Imagine I promised to give you $100 a year from today. How much will you be willing to give me *today* to secure that $100 return a year from today? Well, the simplest answer could be $100. You give me $100 today, and I will return it to you in a year. Actually, the simplest answer would be *nothing.* After all, why should you trust me with your $100, and why trust me for a whole year? After all, a lot can happen to your $100 in a year in my hands. And, besides, if you kept $100 in a risk-free savings account (such as a CD), in a year you would get more than $100, wouldn't you?

And there lies the problem. There are alternatives to giving me $100 in return for the promise of getting it back in a year, and there is risk associated with giving it to *me.* After all, I am not to be trusted with your money. There is likelihood that I will take it and run, or simply lose it and not be able to pay you back, and you would never see your $100 again.

Hence the term Net Present Value: a promise of $100 in the future is worth less than the value of $100 today. Today's value of $100 is called the Net Present Value of that $100. In order to convert the future value to the present value you need to apply a *discount rate*. If a bank is willing to give you 5% annual interest rate on your investments and the federal government is willing to guarantee your funds so they are completely *risk-free*, then the promise of $100 in a year is only worth $95.24 *today* (add 5% to $95.24 and you get $100). In other words, the NPV of $100 a year from now at a 5% discount rate is $95.24. What is the value of that $100 if promised *three* years from now? It is $86.38 today (if you deposit $86.38 and are guaranteed 5% interest rate annually, at the end of three years you should get $100).

But the discount rate we considered here only assumes a federally guaranteed, risk-free interest rate of alternative investments. Should you give me $86.38 today if I promise to return $100 to you in three years? Not really. Why? Because giving it to me is *not* risk free. You don't know if I will have $100 to return in three years. In three years there is a better likelihood that I will take the money and run. So, how about $50? Would you be willing to give me $50 today if I promise to give you $100 in three years? Obviously, there is no risk-free alternative with such a return. So, what say you?

To answer this question you need to calculate NPV with a higher discount rate, one that incorporates the risk. Maybe 20%? A $100 promised in three years with a discount rate of 20% has a Net

Present Value of $57.87. A $100 promised in five years with a discount rate of 30% (higher risk) will have a Net Present Value of less than $27.

Now, the purpose of this part was not to turn you into an economist, accountant, a banker, or an investment advisor. It is just to explain the concept of Net Present Value, and that $100 return promised in five years have less value, much less value, than $100 promised today. You will soon see where I'm going with this.

***

The second concept is taken from the field of *management*, and deals with management's attention to the financial results of the current quarter rather than long-term strategy and investment.

When I worked for Texas Instruments, I had profit-and-loss responsibility for a business unit—making me what is typically referred to as "general manager"—with revenue of just under 100 million dollars. At TI, every year around September-October, all business units set priorities for the coming year. In late 2004, as our team was reviewing the priorities for 2005, something bothered me. There was a "grow the revenue 20% in 2005" priority line. I couldn't tell what bothered me that day, but later that night it dawned on me (even though, *night* is not supposed to be the time when things *dawn* on you). I saw my manager the next morning and asked her, "Do you know what's missing here? We have to 'grow the revenue 20% next year,' but we aren't to 'grow the revenue 100% in four years.'" Her answer was that the two are one and the same. If we continue to grow the revenue 20% every year, in four years it will grow it 100% (actually, 107%). So what's wrong with the priority of growing the revenue 20% next year? Well, to me the two were completely different. In the technology space (and especially in the semiconductor sector), in order to grow your revenue *next year* you better have the products you need to sell readily available. You cannot develop any new product and expect it to generate revenue next year because product development takes up to *four* years. What you have is "baggage." And if you continue to only focus on growing revenue 20% every year, you will never develop new products. But if your goal is to grow revenue 100% in four years, you can start with almost a clean slate. Nothing is off the table. You have far fewer restrictions and can envision products that were not conceived yet.

The result of the conversation was that I became the Director of Strategy for the group of businesses and successfully pushed for the creation of the USB 3.0 "super-speed" connectivity standard. But that's a topic for another book (This approach is partially covered in my first book, *Bowling with a Crystal Ball*.).

Why was it so hard for me to convince her? Why do managers focus so heavily on short-term results and not long-term success?

I've had the word "strategy" in my last three job titles for more than a decade now. But being a strategist is a tough job because, as I experienced at TI, managers pay attention to the short-term more than the long-term, and strategists do the opposite. Strategists are paid to worry about the future—the *far* future. They don't seem to appreciate the importance of the current quarter (I was often blamed for that.).

Gary Hamel, Professor of Strategy at Stanford University and the University of London, once questioned the short term performance focus of CEOs: "Hire a CEO who is two years under the mandatory retirement age, give him a boatload of stock options, and

     Yoram Solomon

get out of the way. Stock price will go up, but will it generate real wealth?"

The average employment term has dramatically declined over the past 100 years. In 2012, the average employment term was 4.6 years of holding a single job[8], while a century ago most people used to work for only one company throughout a professional lifetime. Proof of this is that, although the average employment term is 4.6 years, it is 10.3 years for employees age 65 or more, (more than half of employees age 55 or higher worked for more than 10 years in one job on average), while 91% of Millennials (born between 1977-1997) expect to stay in a job for less than three years[9]. CEOs are no longer the founders of the companies they lead. Instead, they are "hired guns" who come in, demand very high pay, and promise to turn the company around, quickly. *Harvard Business Review,* in 2013, suggested that the optimal CEO tenure should be 4.8 years for optimal company performance, although quite a few CEOs among the 356 companies surveyed between 2000 and 2010 had tenure of 3 years or less. Shareholders don't have the patience to build companies that will endure forever anymore. They want to see immediate results. So, if I join a company as the new CEO, it is expected from me that the performance will improve in the *first* year, preferably in the first quarter. As CEO, when I'm faced with two investment alternatives, one that will yield 25% return in one year and another that will yield 200% return in four years, I am more likely to choose the first one. After all, with employment terms (especially for CEOs)

---

[8] http://www.bls.gov/news.release/pdf/tenure.pdf
[9] http://www.forbes.com/sites/jeannemeister/2012/08/14/job-hopping-is-the-new-normal-for-millennials-three-ways-to-prevent-a-human-resource-nightmare/

becoming so short, what is the probability that I will still be employed with this company to see the returns on a long-term investment and the benefits that come from them? The expenses, though, will definitely occur during my term, and these expenses will adversely affect my short-term benefits. So I might as well make an investment in which I will see the benefit.

What does all of that have to do with *The Worst Diet Ever*? You'll soon see, but for now, let's just agree that in corporate America (where most people work) attention is given more to *short-term results and efforts* than long-term benefits. And this is why "grow the revenue 20% next year" was more important than "grow the revenue 100% in four years."

***

This need for instant gratification is also referred to in Behavioral Economics as "Hyperbolic Time Discounting[10]," in which the immediately available reward has a disproportionate effect on preferences, to the point of reversing a decision that was just made *not* to get that reward. For an applicable example, right before dinner you make a commitment to yourself, for the benefit of your own long-term health, *not* to eat dessert, but as soon as that dessert is in front of you, the immediate availability causes you to reverse your original decision. The future—far future—of the value and benefit are somewhat unclear, whereas the cost of the immediate effort is crystal clear. This phenomenon was supported in the research of authors who procrastinated while writing books and, then, imposed deadlines on themselves. However, as those deadlines grew nearer,

---

[10] http://cowles.econ.yale.edu/P/cd/d17a/d1719.pdf

　　　　　　　　　　　　　　　　　Yoram Solomon

authors' assessments of cost (time and effort to write) grew higher, while the benefits of completing the books (fame, royalties) became increasingly unclear[11]. Note to self: Finish writing this book!

Oh, and you are probably wondering what ever happened to the third concept? Well, you will find it in the next chapter.

---

[11] Akerlof, G.A. (1991). Procrastination and obedience. American Economic Review, 81, 1–19

It's not that long-term health is not important. It is very important. The problem is that it is so far into the future, which makes it hard to balance against the immediate, albeit much less important, pleasures of present life.

2.

MOTIVATION

The third concept needed to explain my theory, as it is put into practice, is taken from the field of Psychology, and known as Intrinsic vs. Extrinsic Motivation.

Between 2008 and 2010 I worked diligently on my dissertation, which was the last requirement to get my Doctoral degree, which I finally received in 2010 (Although, I have to disclaim, as my then nine year old Shira said: "He's a Doctor, but not the useful kind"). I have a Doctoral degree in Organization and Management, and my research was in the area of creativity in organizations. Without getting into too much detail (again, a topic for another book, which I'm sure I'll finish one day), I compared factors affecting employee creativity in startup companies versus mature companies.

The bottom line is that employees are more creative when they are appropriately motivated to be so. Research, done before mine, distinguished between two type of motivation: *intrinsic* (internal) and *extrinsic* (external)[12]. Extrinsic motivation was defined as external to the task environment, while intrinsic motivation is contained within the task itself and the person conducting the task. Extrinsic motivation is easier for management to influence than intrinsic motivation because it is easier to measure and implement. It is

---

[12] Benabou, R., & Tirole, J. (2003). Intrinsic and extrinsic motivation. Review of economic studies, 70(244), 489-520.

made mostly of financial rewards, incentives and promotions and, in general, *contingent* rewards (contingent upon reaching certain milestones or otherwise measurable variables of success or interest).

However, Professor Teresa Amabile of the Harvard Business School, considered one of the gurus in the area of creativity in organizations[13], claimed that *intrinsic* motivation, originating from the task itself, has a much more *positive* influence on creativity, and my own research, as well as generally accepted, supported that.

I came across one of the more fascinating studies in motivation when I worked on my research. It was published in the 1939 book *Management and the Worker*, written by Roethlisberger and Dickson. I remember ordering the book online at the Ann Arbor University Library, not believing that the book, although listed as "in stock," would ever arrive. I remember the feeling of holding a book printed in 1939 in my hands. The book was published as World War II had just started. This book described an experiment conducted at the Hawthorne Works Western Electric company facility. The surprising results of the experiment are known as the "Hawthorne Effect" and are considered foundational to the study of workplace motivation. The real purpose of the experiment was to study the effect of lighting level on productivity. The researcher's hypothesis was that as lighting levels were lowered, the workers' productivity would decline. Sounds simple and logical. Isn't it? However, the results showed exactly the opposite and, for decades, puzzled the original researchers of that study and those that came after. Why would the level of productivity *increase* with lower lighting?

---

[13] Amabile, T. M. (1998). How to kill creativity. Harvard Business Review, 76(5), 76-87.

Yoram Solomon

Eventually, the mystery was solved. It originated at the way that studies are conducted. In order to learn the effect of a certain factor (independent variable) on an outcome (dependent variable), the test subjects (the participants) are divided into two groups: one is called the *control* group, and the other is called the *test* group. Both are subject to exactly the same conditions and environment, except for the changes in the independent, controlled variable of interest, and the outcomes from both groups are compared to test the effect of the independent variable on the dependent variable. However, the control group used during the Hawthorne experiment (the one with the regular lighting) was *not informed* of the experiment, while the test group (the one with the lower lighting) *was* informed. While the control group workers worked as they always have, the workers in the test group felt they were observed and seemingly felt it necessary to *prove* their ability to produce. They worked extra hard to show better productivity, even in lower lighting conditions. Team spirit was created. Workers helped other workers more than in the control group, who were not aware of the ongoing experiment and comparison. The knowledge that they were being scrutinized and analyzed gave the test group workers the motivation to perform better—so much that they performed better than the control group, the one with better lighting. What researchers missed initially was the difference in the *knowledge* about the test. The knowledge of the test significantly impacts results.

The Hawthorne effect is a perfect example of *intrinsic* motivation, where people are motivated by something rising from the task itself and not *external* to it. There were no bonuses promised, only the knowledge that one team outperformed the other.

⁎⁎⁎

On September 12, 1962, President John F. Kennedy gave one of the most inspiring speeches of that decade at the stadium of Rice University in Houston, Texas[14]. Facing Soviet early successes in space, the President inspired the nation to put a man on the moon before the end of the decade: "We choose to go to the moon. We choose to go to the moon in this decade and do the other things, not because they are easy, but because they are *hard*, because that goal will serve to organize and measure the best of our energies and skills, because that challenge is one that we are willing to accept, one we are unwilling to postpone, and one which we intend to win, and the others, too."

This, again, is a wonderful example of intrinsic motivation. The motivation to put a man on the moon is driven by the need to *prove* to the Soviets (and to the US nation itself) that we *can* do hard things. It is driven by the *pride* from success against strong hurdles. Not because of any financial, economical, or other benefits, it is pure intrinsic motivation. And it worked.

But I'm not asking you to put a man on the moon, nor am I asking you to beat the performance of another team. My success in losing 32 pounds was not equivalent to the success of the Apollo 11 program—not by a long stretch. And there is probably no clear and present danger to your life if you don't lose 80 pounds right now, as in Joe's story that comes next.

***

---

[14] http://er.jsc.nasa.gov/seh/ricetalk.htm

Yoram Solomon

I have a hobby. I actually have several hobbies, but this one will play a significant role throughout this book. I always loved aviation. Ever since I was very young, I visited every aviation museum I could and read every aviation book and magazine I found. I knew almost everything there was to know about aviation. At about thirteen, I joined a model aviation club in Israel and started building free-flying sailplanes from plans using Balsa wood and silk paper. It took a long time, and they were not as fun to fly as radio controlled airplanes that I saw others build and fly. Those, of course, involved the use of liquid (read: smelly and messy) fuel with loud internal combustion engines. The first time I got a chance (when I was in my twenties) to fly such a plane that belonged to a friend for a short while, I love it but never owned one then. They cost a lot of money, they smell, they are messy, and they need a runway to take off from and land on. I didn't have access to any of those when I was thirteen, and not much even when I was in my twenties. However, after I joined Interphase Corporation as the Vice President of Corporate Strategy in 2008, the CEO, a radio controlled airplane builder and flyer himself, encouraged me to enter the hobby—again. Except, this time I had the money. I had a much bigger house than I ever owned (or lived in) before, where I could house this hobby (of course, at that point I didn't know that I will at some point, own more than 30 airplanes), despite my wife's protest. What also helped was the evolution of electric power in this hobby, which eliminated the smelly and messy part of it. So I bought the first plane, which was a trainer. Then I bought the second one and third one and more and more. I love this hobby. It has an important place in my life. This hobby is not stress free at all. Flying a ten-pound, 130 miles per hour jet for five minutes can be stressful. But it is also enjoyable, and it breaks you away from everything else on your mind. Soon, I became so involved with the hobby that every day I would buy something (it could be a servo, screw, wire, wheel, or even a whole new airplane), build something, or fly something. Every day.

And then I discovered the hobby shop, and I became a "regular" there. I got to know all the sales associates in that store. Including Joe. Joe is a retired police officer who was not a very pleasant person to buy from before I got to know him. I'm sure his life made him the way he was, but it wasn't pleasant to ask him for help. It felt like asking would be to interrupt him. He was cordial, but just not as inviting as you would expect a salesperson to be. Joe was about my height but seemed to be a bit heavier than me. I never thought much of his weight, until that day.

I came to buy something, and all of a sudden I saw Joe, or someone that looked somewhat like Joe minus fifty pounds or so. His face was much thinner.

"Joe?" I hesitated.

"Yes? How can I help you?" It was him. The tone was more like "What do you want from me now?" I saw what chemotherapy did to people. The loss of appetite and the effects of the drugs on the body looked just like Joe. So I assumed.

"Are you OK?"

"Yes, I am."

Well, I was puzzled now.

"You lost some weight?"

"Eighty pounds." OK, more than fifty.

"How come?"

And then he told me an interesting story. I don't think Joe was drinking much, and I guess it was the effect of body fat that his liver couldn't break down anymore. He went to his doctor for a regular checkup, and the doctor asked him, pretty bluntly, if he could identify a relative who could donate a piece of liver to him because his liver was just about done. When Joe asked for an alternative to a liver transplant, the doctor told him that he had to immediately lose a dramatic amount of weight in order to reduce the level of fat in his body. You see, when we think about dieting, we think about the long-term health consequences, but we don't think about the need for a liver transplant right now. In the next several months, Joe had all the incentive he needed, and he lost 80 pounds. It was a combination of eating only vegetables, working out intensively, and many other things, I'm sure. Joe needed exactly what his doctor gave him: *motivation.*

I didn't tell you Joe's story to talk about him, his attitude, or anything else. If there is one thing I learned in life, it is not to judge people. So, I'm not judging. I learned a few things about Joe's life that could explain a lot about his attitude toward life and to people. I respect Joe, and his story inspired me. I can't say that we became friends as I was, after all, just a passing-through customer.

Joe's story is, again, a story of *intrinsic* motivation. His motivation came from the direct results of losing weight. However, it is very important to realize that the benefits Joe perceived from his drastic diet were extreme ("*start looking for a liver donor…*") and very immediate ("*…now!*"), and did not have to be discounted. The benefits to *you* from the diet you need, for which you were willing to spend your money, although as important, are not as *immediate* and will, thus, need to be discounted.

***

Alex is a member of my Rotary club. One day we sat at the same table for lunch during our regular weekly meeting and, when he heard that I was writing a book about weight loss, he immediately jumped:

"I lost 55 pounds!"

What he told me later seemed very consistent with what I describe in this book, so I scheduled a lunch meeting with him to hear his story.

Alex was a skinny child. He weighed 140 pounds when he graduated from high school and 155 when he graduated from college. Then he started bodybuilding and put on a lot of muscle weight, to the point he weighed 260 pounds. So far, this was OK. A 260 pound bodybuilder doesn't look like a 260 pounds, well, *fat* person. And he was fine with that. But then he stopped working out. Sure, he knew he had hypertension (high blood pressure) and that he really needed to lose weight, but that's a long-term health concern—not as important as the food in front of him or the exercise he started avoiding. Alex got married and had two girls, while much of his 260 pounds turned from muscle into fat. Then, one day in 2012, just about the same time I was interviewed on NBC, his 7 year old daughter said to him:

"Daddy, you're fat. People will make fun of you, and *I don't want you to die.*"

Yoram Solomon

Unless you are a parent, you don't know how powerful those words can be when they are coming from your 7 year old daughter.

Alex started losing weight. He worked out (he currently rides his bike for an hour every morning, covering about 12 miles daily). He uses a (free) app called *MyFitnessPal*[15] that helps him count calories all day, so he can live within a daily calorie "budget." He was using this app as we ordered lunch so he would know what to choose. He didn't touch the Shiner Bock Beer bread, or at least not until he found that the bread loaf only had 200 calories, at which point he decided to eat half the loaf. Alex lost 55 pounds. The only reason he didn't lose more was that his wife told him he shouldn't. His daughter's words still echo in his head every day (two years later), but my guess is that the main driving force to keep him "on target" is that the new lifestyle he adopted became a *habit.*

***

In my survey, I asked about people's motivation to lose and keep weight off. Of the four options I gave for that question, the most effective one was, "An immediate health risk or life threat that needed to be taken care of now". Like Joe, 80% of those who indicated they started losing weight due to a clear and present danger to their lives managed to lose a significant amount of weight, and 67% of them managed to keep most of the weight off for at least three months at the time of participating in my research. But if you are not immediately threatened, you will not have this type of motivation. After getting some feedback from a few of my participants, I realized that there could have been another category, although it might have

---

[15] http://www.myfitnesspal.com/

been hidden under the "immediate health risk or life threat" and that was a *breakdown*. A few of my participants (they reached out to me after responding to the survey) simply reached a point in which they just didn't like themselves anymore. They were tired of what they looked like or how they felt, and the last pound gained was also the last straw. These respondents simply *broke down*. That's what happened to Alex when his daughter said, "People will laugh at you, and I don't want you to die." That is a pretty powerful motivator, which would probably have as strong an effect on weight loss as your doctor instructing you to find a liver donor. However, I'm not suggesting that in order to get motivated to lose weight you should somehow induce a breakdown. This is only to explain the effectiveness of this motivator. If you have experienced one, though, then I hope this book will help you put it to positive use.

***

One thing I heard over and over again in the context of weight loss is that you need *discipline* to lose weight. It seems to me that this is somewhat stating the obvious. You need to do certain things at certain times—consistently. That's discipline. I looked up the many dictionary definitions for the word "discipline," and the one I found to be most appropriate to use in this context is: "behavior and order maintained by training and control[16]." You need to maintain control to be disciplined throughout the effort required for weight loss. But in this book I'm not going to make you feel bad for your lack of discipline and self-control, because that's not really what you need. What you need first is *motivation* so that you can be disci-

---

[16] http://dictionary.reference.com/browse/discipline?s=t

　　　　　　　　　　　　　　　　　Yoram Solomon

plined in your weight loss. I'm not splitting hair here. Those are two different things.

This is not a book about weight loss. This is a book about creating the *motivation* to lose weight. The term *motivation* will be used abundantly throughout the book, so it only begs that I explain the word. The dictionary definition of *motivation* is almost useless: "providing a reason to act in a certain way[17]." However, the text-book[18] definition of *motivation* starts with two general questions: (1) what causes behavior? And (2) why does behavior vary in its intensity?

The first question (What causes behavior?) is further expanded into five secondary questions:

- Why does a certain behavior start?
- Once begun, why is the behavior sustained over time?
- Why is the behavior directed toward some goals, yet away from other?
- Why does the behavior change its direction? and—
- Why does the behavior stop?

To frame it according to the textbook definition, the purpose of my book is to explain *how* and to help find the motivation *to*:

- Start the behaviors required to lose weight;
- Continue those behaviors over a long period of time;
- Direct those behaviors towards the goal of losing weight;

---

[17] http://dictionary.reference.com/browse/motivation?s=t
[18] Reeve, J. "Understanding Motivation and Emotion", 5th Edition, Wiley, Hoboken, NJ, 2009

- Prevent those behaviors from changing direction;
- Prevent those behaviors from stopping; and—
- Assuring that those behaviors have enough intensity to go through the efforts required to lose weight.

***

Thus far in this chapter I made the case for why intrinsic motivation works *better* than extrinsic one. In my Ph.D. research I found that extrinsic motivation had little to no positive impact on levels of *creativity*. But before we completely give up on extrinsic motivation, let's see if it *ever* works and before we start, let's talk about the candle problem. Yes, it's a real problem[19]. The candle problem is a cognitive performance test, developed by psychologist Karl Duncker and published in 1945. In this test, participants are given a candle, matches, and a box of thumbtacks. The objective is to fix a lit candle on the wall, such that wax will not drip from it onto the floor. Think about it for a second; how would you do it?

The answer is to take the thumbtacks out of their box, use them to fix the box itself to the wall, and then put the lit candle in that box. If you reached that conclusion, you are creative (or at least were at the time of the test) and less affected by "functional fixed-ness" (limiting your imagination to the *normal* use of things, such as the box being used only to hold the thumbtacks).

The next step is to add a factor: perform the test with the thumbtacks provided *outside* the box versus inside the box. When they are outside the box, it is clear to see that the box can be used for

---

[19] http://en.wikipedia.org/wiki/Candle_problem

   Yoram Solomon

other purposes (such as holding the candle) and, thus, more test participants will reach the right solution fast. Not much creativity or complex thought was required in this case.

In 1962, psychologist Sam Glucksberg[20] took this test to the next level by adding another factor: offering a $5 (in 1962 values) to the fastest 25% of those who solved the candle problem, and $20 to those who were the fastest of all. There were, thus, four groups: two groups with the offered incentives and two groups without them. For each there was one group in which the thumbtacks were *inside* the box (requiring more creativity) and one group in which the thumbtacks were *outside* the box (more obvious, requiring less creativity). Glucksberg expected to find that the incentives will *improve* performance regardless of the task/test complexity, but to his surprise he found the opposite: offering the incentives *decreased* performance sometimes.

In 2005, the Federal Reserve Bank of Boston commissioned research to find the impact of contingent pay incentives on productivity and performance[21]. The research was conducted by Dan Ariely (MIT), Uri Gneezy (University of Chicago), George Lowenstein (Carnegie Mellon University), and Nina Mazar (MIT). The experiments were conducted at MIT, the University of Chicago, and rural India. The participants were given six games to play, with varying levels of complexity and varying need for creative thinking. Based on

---

[20] Glucksberg, S. (1962). The influence of strength of drive on functional fixedness and perceptual recognition. Journal of Experimental Psychology, 63 (1), 36-41: http://whywereason.com/2011/09/01/how-misguided-incentives-negatively-affect-productivity-and-well-being/

[21] Ariely, D., U. Gneezy, G. Lowenstein and N. Mazar (2009): "Large Stakes and Big Mistakes," Review of Economic Studies 76, 451-469: http://www.bostonfed.org/economic/wp/wp2005/wp0511.pdf

the results of the games, they were offered incentives (compared to the control groups that were *not* offered any incentives). The highest possible performance rewarded participants a sum equal to a median monthly wage. The results were consistent with those of Glucksberg in 1962: while the performance has improved *with* incentives at the simple tasks, they actually *deteriorated* at the more complex tasks that required creativity. To use the researchers' own words:

> "It now appears that beyond some threshold level, raising incentives may increase motivation to supra-optimal levels and result in perverse effects on performance."

Figure 1 shows the effect that incentives have on simple and complex tasks, as discovered by the abovementioned researchers.

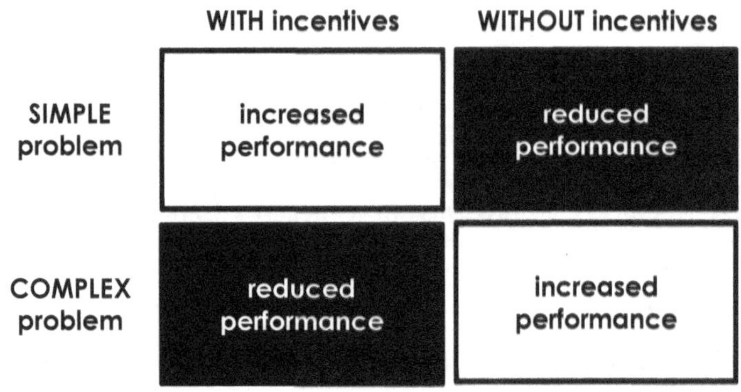

Figure 1: The effect of incentives on performance at different task complexities

As I'm about to continue and describe the core of the theory behind my weight loss motivation, for now just remember the following: *extrinsic* motivation has a *positive* effect on *simple* tasks while it has a *negative* effect on *complex* tasks that require creativity.

Oh, and one more thing: weight loss is a *simple* task. It does not require creativity. It is not rocket science. It only requires *motivation*. And based on the above, *extrinsic* motivation should work here, while intrinsic motivation might not. Let's see.

*****

Around February of 2011, I became fascinated with the Colt 1911 pistol. As its name suggests, this pistol went into service in 1911, even before World War I. It was designed to meet a requirement of the US government. Six companies submitted their designs for a semi-automatic .45 caliber pistol, and the Colt M1911 pistol, designed by John Browning, won the contract after a test in which it fired 6,000 rounds without a single malfunction (can we say that about anything today?). This pistol served during World War I, World War II, the Korean War, the Vietnam War, and every war the US military took part in until it was retired in the early 1990s. I first saw the Colt 1911 "Government" (with the long barrel) through my shooting instructor in Israel in the late 1970s, while I was still in high school. I next saw this pistol in the Sam Peckinpah's 1969 western *The Wild Bunch*, which is set in 1913.

At the same time (around February of 2011), my weight was 223 pounds. I had hard time tying my shoelaces; I didn't like what I looked like, suffered almost constant heartburns, and decided it was time to lose weight. Even before knowing what I know now about motivation, I decided that my health, longevity, and ability to tie my shoelaces were not motivating me enough, so I made a deal with myself: if I got my weight under 205 pounds (losing 18 pounds)—I could buy a Colt 1911. 2011 was a special year for the 1911 because it was the centennial anniversary. A quick look at the Colt website showed that they were going to have two variants of the centennial anniversary model. One was the 1918 model, and the other was a gold-plated collectors-only model, which was three times more expensive. I wanted the 1918 model. It was an exact reproduction of the 1911A1 version manufactured in 1918. It was going to be produced in a very limited production run. I wanted to have one, and it was going to be my incentive to lose weight. After all, weight loss by itself was not a good enough incentive for me. So I started eating less and exercising more. I weighed myself often to see how I was doing. It really only took some two months for me to get up one morning and see that I was just under 205 pounds. Mission accomplished!

And then I set out to buy the 1911 centennial edition. I first drove to the local gun store. They didn't have it but were willing to try to order it for me. But I wanted it *now*. So I then went to the Fort Worth Gun Show, possibly the biggest gun show in North Texas (maybe in all of Texas). I didn't find the gun anywhere. Nobody had it. They all said it was a very limited edition and very hard to find. Some were willing to take my order (and my money) just to see if they could find it for me, but I didn't want to take that risk. A few people told me that the Dallas Market Gun Show was actually bigger than the Fort Worth Gun Show, so I went there too. Nobody had that centennial anniversary model. Then, I started going to smaller gun shows, like the ones in Frisco and Mesquite. But I never found it. I started calling arms dealers, but nobody had the gun. Finally, I called Colt in Hartford, Connecticut to ask them where I could find the gun. The person on the other side of the line started laughing: "Son, this is a limited edition gun. We sold out in 2009!" Two years before they started making it. Apparently there were people more interested in it than I was—much more. And they purchased it long before Colt even decided what the centennial model would be.

OK, so I'm not much of a collector or enthusiast as others were. But I still wanted that piece of history. And it was starting to get hard to stay under 205 pounds, as I really saw this as a one-time effort rather than a sustainable one that I will need to maintain for the rest of my life. Well, there were other models I could get. There was the series 70, which was used during the Vietnam War. There was also the modern series 80 (also called model 1991), with a better safety mechanism (you see, with a pre-series 80 1911, if it has a round in the chamber, and the hammer was not cocked, and it fell on the floor and hit the hammer first—that bullet will fire, and could completely ruin your day). Both are still in production and much more reasonably priced, as not one of them is the centennial anniversary model. So I decided to get a series 80 gun. I drove to the next Fort Worth Gun Show and bought it. Less than a month later my weight was back above 220 pounds.

What happened? First of all, it became very clear that a motivator having nothing to do with health or losing weight was much more effective than any motivation related to my health. This was an *extrinsic* motivator! However, losing weight over a period of two months did not create new diet and exercise habits. It was a significant effort over a period of time, but once the milestone was reached, it was over. You apply different strengths (psychological and emotional, rather than physical) to get you over a *hurdle* than you do if you need to *sustain* an effort. You look at it as a hill that you need to climb, where as soon as you reach the summit, it becomes downhill from there. You could probably achieve a more significant weight loss over a short period of time if you knew that at some point you could stop than if you knew you needed to continue with the same effort for—let's face it—the rest of your life. I was always curious to understand how competitors on NBC's "The Biggest Loser" could lose more than 10 pounds a week. It's simple: they knew that after they won the game, it was over. This is true for every effort. But this is also why less than a month later my weight was back above 220 pounds.

In my survey, the participants who indicated that they lost weight as a result of a *milestone* incentive—"I promised myself that if I reach a milestone weight, I would reward myself with something (example: buy a new car)"—have a high success rate in losing weight (67% of them lost significant weight) but had the worst rate in keeping the weight off. Only 30% managed to keep most of the weight off for more than 3 months. 70% of them gained all of it (or more) back.

A clear and present danger to your life is the most effective motivator to lose weight. A milestone external motivator would be effective in losing weight but not in keeping it off for the rest of your life, and intrinsic motivators, well, they simply don't work.

3.

THE WEIGHT LOSS DILEMMA

And with that, I think you are ready to discover how to motivate yourself to lose weight and keep it off for the rest of your life. Take a few minutes to answer this question for yourself: *Why* do I want to lose weight? Stop reading for a few minutes. Take a piece of paper and write the answer to the question. Now keep reading. If I was a gambling man, I would bet that your reasons include some combination of the following:

- I want to feel better
- I want to live longer
- I want to be healthy
- I want to cut down on my medications
- I want to see my daughters get married
- I want to tie my shoes without holding my breath
- I want to look better

Well, all of those are intrinsic-internal motivators. And if I relied on creativity and productivity theories, they should have been much stronger than any extrinsic-external motivators. But we already know that. Don't we?

Maybe this is a good time to put the terms *intrinsic* and *extrinsic* motivation in the context of health and weight loss. Intrinsic motivators, those that are "within the task" (of losing weight), are the positive benefits of dieting and exercising. They can be any of the statements listed above and more. However, extrinsic motivators are those that have nothing to do with weight loss, such as buying that Colt 1911, or anything else that is not a benefit directly resulting from losing weight.

There is one common thread to all the intrinsic motivators to lose weight. None of them has an *immediate* benefit (except in an extreme case as Joe's). If I lose weight, I will feel better. But it will take *time*— maybe months, even years. I will look better, but even that will take time. I will live longer, but, let's face it, right now I don't feel like I'm about to die any time soon. Joe felt the *immediate* threat of a potential liver transplant ("or you die"), but you and I don't. I'm sure we all know someone close who died of a heart attack (my father did) or a stroke, which could be the result of being overweight, poor blood pressure control, or high cholesterol, but *we* feel invincible; this will never happen to us. I need to lose weight for a *long* period of time before I can secure all those long-term "will not happen to me anyway" seemingly intangible benefits of losing weight. So we apply a "discount rate" on those, and we get a pretty low Net Present Value of those benefits (ha! Now you know why I explained that term).

And there are costs to losing weight. You have to give up food you like. You have to give up 30 minutes you could stay in bed longer and instead exercise (not to mention shower, you could easily spend another 10 minutes there). The dessert looks really good. I'm not going to be the only person who doesn't eat ice cream with everyone! (Yes, peer pressure does play a role here).

There is no doubt that the long-term benefit of losing weight outweighs (no pun intended, yet well-played) the short-term benefits of eating *what* you like, *when* you like it, and engaging in fun activities instead of exercising. The weight loss benefits outweigh the short-term pleasures by much!

However, once you apply that discount rate, the Net Present Value of the long-term benefits from weight loss pales in comparison to the immediate gratification and short-term benefits from *not* losing weight—hence, why diets fail. You weigh (again, accidental pun) the Net Present Value of the long-term intrinsic motivator (living longer, feeling good, even looking good) against the immediate gratification and weight loss loses (I can't help myself, those puns just keep on coming!) every time.

It's funny, but I can actually quantify this economically. Let's assume that my health 25 years from now (I will be 75, so this makes sense) is worth one million dollars to me. This is the kind of sum that you could put into a life insurance policy, so maybe that's what my life is worth. On the other hand, eating that high-sugar dessert is worth $100 to me now (not that it costs $100—it's *worth* that much to me, and since it costs less—I buy it). Let's also say that the discount rate I apply to that value is 33% annually (after all, there are risks in this "investment"). The Net Present Value of my million dollar age-75 life is $40 today: less than $100. I know those numbers are only numbers, and I know we are not putting dollar values on life or immediate gratification, but our minds (and stomachs) make this comparison every time we need to decide whether to eat something that is not healthy or skip a workout. Just like I said at my July 2012 interview on The TODAY show at NBC: "I know what I *can* and *cannot* eat, I know what I have to do, I just don't have the motivation." If I asked you today if you know what you needed to do to lose weight, I bet you would. You might be following a diet that someone recommended, you know you need to work out, so it's not a matter of knowledge. You are not dumb. It's a matter of motivation.

This always reminds me of a statement that Shrek said to Donkey (from the movie *Shrek*, 2001). Both of them were hanging upside down in a jail pit, and Donkey complained: "What about my Miranda rights? You're supposed to say, 'You have the right to remain silent.' Nobody said I have the right to remain silent!" to which Shrek answered: "Donkey, you *have* the right to remain silent. What you lack is the *capacity.*"

We don't lack the *knowledge* to lose weight. What we lack is the *capacity* to do something with that knowledge—the motivation.

***

Let me put this in perspective and in the context of weight loss for long-term health and discuss the motivation dilemma and how this book proposes to solve it. The first premise is that we do (or do not do) things based on a simple cost-benefit analysis. You can compare cost to benefit because they both have *value.* We buy something only if the value we believe to *get* from it is higher than the value we assign to the money we have to *spend* on it. If the value of the benefit is higher than that of the cost, we will do it. If the benefit is lower than the cost, we will simply *not* do it. The farther they are from each other, the clearer the decision is. If the benefit is *much* higher than the cost (or effort)—we will *definitely* do it. If the benefit is *much* lower than the perceived cost (or effort), we will *definitely* not expend that effort. It's really *that* simple.

***

                                                   Yoram Solomon

Figure 2 shows that your long-term health brings more value to you than the effort required with weight loss and, specifically, a healthy diet and exercise. In fact, if I asked you, I'm betting you would say that the benefits of your long-term health are *much* more important to you than the effort required to achieve it through diet and exercise. 67% of the respondents to my survey described their long-term health and/or well-being as the main motivation for their weight loss efforts.

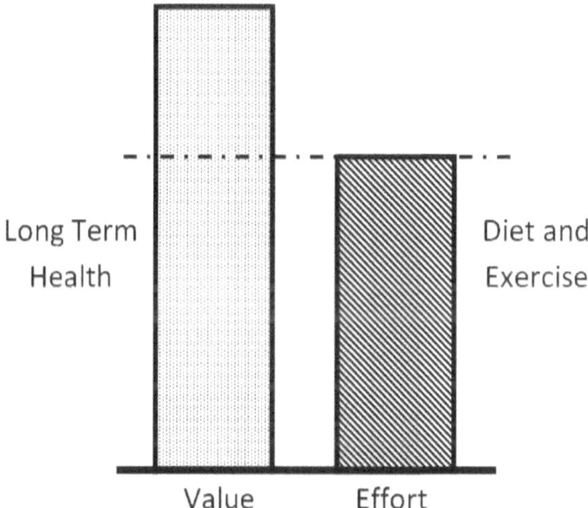

Figure 2: Long-term health vs. diet and exercise effort

But if this is the case, why are we still not willing to make the effort? 83% of those participants in my survey who wanted to lose weight and were motivated by their long-term health actually lost *some* weight, but only 22% of them lost a significant amount of weight (more than 20 lb.), and while 57% of those who lost weight kept most of it off for more than 3 months after losing it, only 29%

kept it off for more than a year. Here is where the Net Present Value concept (from economics and finance) comes into play. Your long-term health is, as its name suggests, a *long-term* issue. As Figure 3 shows, the long-term health is far out into the future (in the back). When a "discount rate" is applied to it to show the Net Present Value of that long-term health, you see a much lower value *today* (in the front). As a result, the present value of your long-term health benefit is *lower* than the cost-effort associated with the diet and exercise required to gain and maintain the long-term health. This is the *long-term health-weight loss motivation dilemma.*

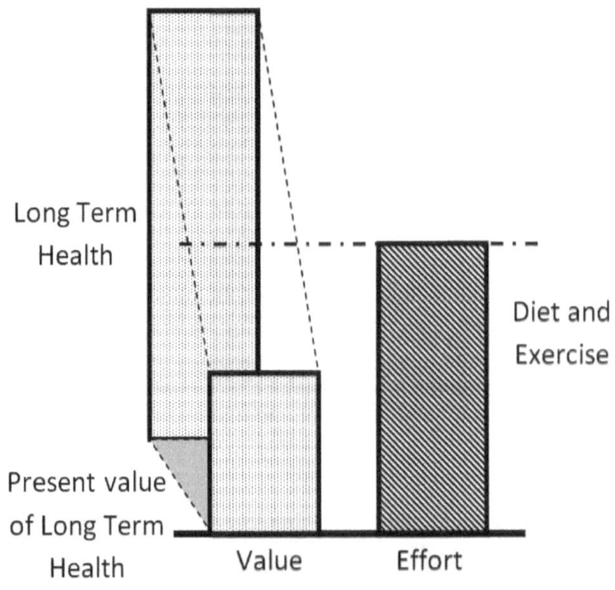

Figure 3: The present value of long-term health

And how do we solve it? Well, this is *exactly* what this book is about. In general terms, as Figure 4 shows, we will add a *present extrinsic*-external motivation factor that, combined with the present

Yoram Solomon

value of the long-term health benefit, will provide *higher* value than the cost-effort required for diet and exercise. Why do I call it extrinsic? Because the benefits it provides have nothing to do with long-term health (at least not directly) or are a natural consequence of the effort, but will nevertheless still be providing value *today*. However, an important element of that motivator is that it has to be, just like my long-term health (or the Net Present Value of it), a *direct* reward depending on, resulting from, and contingent upon the diet and exercise. Except that, unlike your health, the cause-and-effect relationship between the effort and that reward (the extrinsic motivator) is not natural. It is man-made.

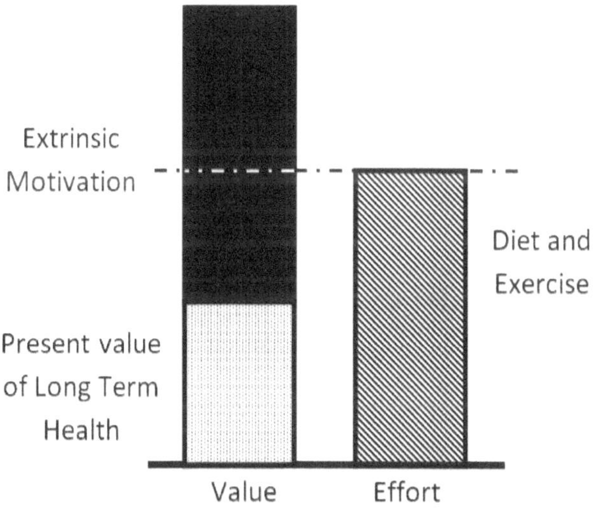

Figure 4: Adding extrinsic motivation

The following chapters will describe and suggest how to develop such motivation. But the question then becomes: do we *forever* need to have this extrinsic motivator in play? The answer is actually *no*. As we engage in diet and exercise, they become less of a chore.

They require less effort. They become more natural. We need to think less about them. They become *habits.* Figure 5 shows that the effort required for diet and exercise is lower over time due to the effect of the creation of new habits. It doesn't happen overnight. The effort gradually, over a long period of time, is reduced. Figure 5 shows that the effort is lower than before but still higher than the perceived benefit of the present value of your long-term health alone. You still need the extrinsic motivator but less so.

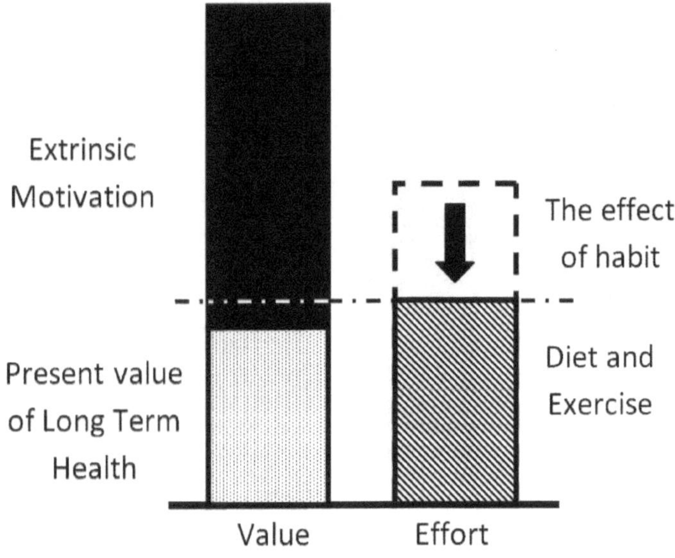

Figure 5: The effect of habits on lowering the effort

However, the effort continues to decline, as diet and exercise become habits, and Figure 6 shows that at some point the effort becomes lower than the perceived Net Present Value of your long-term health. At that point you don't need the extrinsic motivator anymore. You broke the motivation dilemma cycle!

                                        Yoram Solomon

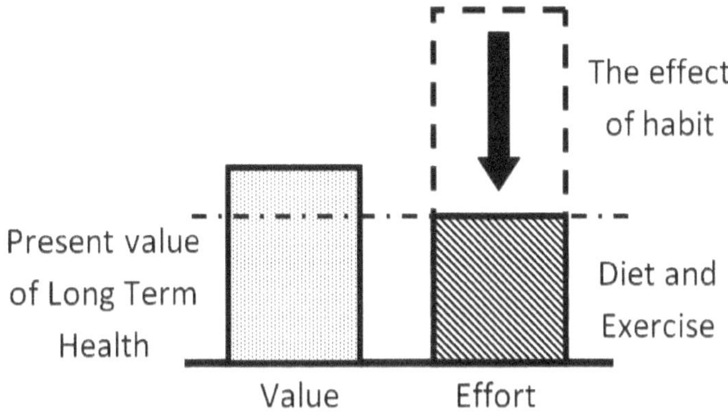

Figure 6: Over time, the effect of habit can be enough to eliminate the need for extrinsic motivation at all!

And that is the core of my theory. I just finished explaining why we have such hard time committing to the discipline of healthy nutrition and physical exercise. It's simple: all you have to do is add an effective external motivator. Let's move on from the *why* to the *how*.

***

In July 2012, once I figured it out, I sent the following email to my wife and my daughters, so it got documented:

Girls,

I need your help. I want to lose weight, and I've been trying for a long time, but couldn't lose weight. For the past 6 months I've been meeting with a dietician, who was supposed to help me lose weight. So, I started with her at 218 lb., and today I was 236 lb.... I gained 18 lb.... I just love to eat so much, and I don't like to work out.

My Doctor said that I have to lose weight. He didn't specifically say that I was at danger, but I suspect I'm not too far from it.

So, why can't I lose weight? Because I need motivation, and I don't have any. In fact, a couple of years ago, I really wanted to buy something, and I made a deal with myself that until I lose 18 lb. (from 223 to 205)—I will not be able to buy that thing. So, guess what? I lost 18lb. Exactly. Then I bought that thing, and then I gained all the weight back.

So, I thought about what would motivate me, and realized that perhaps the one area that can motivate me the most is my RC hobby. I'm thinking about how to tie the hobby to motivation. Also, the motivation needs to have something to do not only with reaching a certain weight goal, but actually staying there. Finally, the motivation doesn't count if I don't make a commitment that I can't break. This is where you come in. I don't need you to remind me all the time that I need to eat less, or work out more. All I need is for you to know that the commitment that I'm making is to you, and that if I don't meet that commitment—you will be disappointed in me. I can't simply say "Who cares? I'll just break my commitment." Because the last thing I want to do is break a commitment to you.

So, here is the commitment and the consequences. While my weight was 236 at the dietician's office, it was really 228 at home (I guess I'm wearing 8lb of cloths). My goals are:

1. *In July 2012, keep my weight below 228 lb.*

2. *After 8/1/2012, keep my weight below 222 lb.*

Yoram Solomon

3. *After 9/1/2012, keep my weight below 216 lb.*

4. *After 10/1/2012, keep my weight below 210 lb.*

5. *After 11/1/2012, keep my weight below 205 lb.*

6. *After 12/31/2012, keep my weight below 200 lb.*

This means that I need to lose 28lb in 6 months. This can be done, and is not too aggressive.

The consequences: whenever my weight is higher than the "allowed" weight for that time, I will not be able to go flying RC airplanes, buy anything for RC airplanes, or build RC airplanes, until I get my weight below the "allowed" weight for that time. If I break this rule, and either buy, fly, or build RC airplanes while my weight is ABOVE the "allowed" weight for that time—I will be breaking a commitment to YOU. Not just to me.

Now, note one thing: if I cannot keep my weight under the allowed weight for the time, while I cannot fly, buy, or build—I will be able to go watch. Why? Because watching will only provide more motivation. Imagine me watching RC planes but not able to build, fly, or buy? It would be terrible! It will only motivate me more.

So, do we have a deal?

Daddy/Roma.

Since I didn't edit this letter before including it here, I feel that it is only fair that I explain something. It is clear why I signed this letter with "Daddy", but not so clear why I also signed it as "Roma."

Well, let's just leave this between my wife and I, but if you see us in public together, and you hear her calling me "Roma," know that she still loves me.

As I explain this method, I want you to note the following elements of the plan included in the email to my daughters:

- I needed to lose 28 pounds. I stretched it over a period of 6 months (even though I thought I could lose it in one month). I gave myself two months to lose the last 5 pounds—the easiest period, which prepared me to maintain my target weight.
- I tied the weight loss to my *hobby*, on a *daily* basis, since my hobby had daily activities (buying, building, or flying). Every day I didn't meet my goals, I was prevented from the reward associated with the hobby. This also forced me to weigh myself on a daily basis. If I missed my goal one day, then I missed the reward, but could still catch up and achieve it the following day.
- The steps were monthly, which made them easier to remember. I didn't have to look up my exact weight limit (in tenths of a pound) every day. I only needed to remember the weight limit for the current month.
- I made the promise to my *daughters*. I entered a deal with them. They were my "enforcers." If I had made the deal with myself, the risk would have been too high that I would "cut corners" and break my promise to myself.

Adding an external motivator to the Net Present Value of your long-term health, with a reward contingent upon weight-loss, will be enough to help you create new healthy habits.

4.

SETTING GOALS, CHANGING HABITS

Whenever I watched (and admittedly, not very often) NBC's "The Biggest Loser," I saw people lose over ten pounds in one week. Sure, there were weeks they would actually gain weight, but in general they lost quite a bit. In my opinion, the diet regimes (between less food and more, much more workout) they used were too drastic and not sustainable. My fear was that if I wanted to lose 32 pounds in one month I could, but then I would have to scale my efforts back. Exactly how far back was not clear, and then I would have to develop new habits.

***

Getting to work every day is a highly complex operation. You need to remember where the car is. Take the car keys. Walk to the car. Unlock the door. Enter from the driver's side (the left side of the car, unless you are in England, Australia, Japan, or any other British colony, in which case you are in for a surprise if you enter from the left). Put on your seat belt. Put the car keys in the ignition switch. Make sure the parking brake is engaged. Make sure the car is in neutral (if it has a manual gear) or "Park" (if automatic). Turn the ignition switch to the "on" position. Then continue to the momentary starting point. Hold it there only until you hear the engine start. Then, release and let it return to the "on" position. I could go on and on, but you get the point. Driving a car is a very complex operation. In fact, if we have to think about everything we do when we drive a car, every time we drive, we would probably pretty soon quit and start taking the bus.

Let's talk about the bus ride, then. Before you leave home, you need to make sure that you know the bus schedule. Take the right amount of change for the bus ride. Calculate the distance between your home and the bus station, and compare it with the bus schedule. Leave home such that you will arrive at the bus station two minutes ahead of the bus. Then look to the left (unless you are in any of the British colonies, in which you will look to the right, because those buses simply don't come from the left there), and wait for the bus. When the bus arrives, wait for it to open the front doors. Then, climb in and offer the driver the change you prepared before you left home. OK, this is not much simpler than driving a car.

Do you think about all those things whenever you drive a car or ride the bus? You don't. But you still do them perfectly in a repeatable way every morning. Every little mistake can kill you. Yet, you don't make mistakes. I bet you can't describe your drive to work this morning in the level of detail because your brain was not consciously thinking about those details. It was as if it was on "autopilot." We are lazy. So are our brains. They constantly look for ways to save effort[22]. This shortcut is called *habits*. The first time you drove a car, it was far from being a habit. You had to think about every little detail. However, after a while you stopped thinking about it. It became automatic. It became a habit. When you move to a new office, you initially have to think about the *road.* Not so much about how to

---

[22] Duhigg, Charles, The Power of Habit: Why we do what we do in life and business

Yoram Solomon

drive the car, but really only how different is this new road than the old one. But after a few months, this becomes a habit as well.

This concept is even known in the area of Management. Peter Drucker, considered one of the gurus in the art of management wrote a chapter (titled *Effective Decisions* in his 1966 book *The Effective Executive*, suggesting when to make decisions and when to create rules. According to Drucker, when the environment and circumstances change all the time, you need to make different appropriate decisions, but when the environment and circumstances remain constant, we need a shortcut—we need *rules* that we could follow without spending the mental effort required to make a decision. Just like habits.

***

There are several advantages to habits. First of all, they work on things that are repetitive. Things you do over and over, in exactly the same way, every time. Guess what? Those tend to get boring pretty quickly, and if we had to think about them every time we did them, we probably wouldn't. We would simply abandon them. And those might be habits important for us!

When I started working for Texas Instruments, we lived in Sunnyvale, California, in the heart of Silicon Valley. But my office was up in wine country, in Santa Rosa. The commute was 99.9 miles each way, every day. Don't get me wrong. I am not complaining about that commute. It was the most beautiful commute ever. I drove up highway 280, between the mountains and the bay, drove up 19th Avenue in San Francisco, and then over the Golden Gate Bridge (in fact, the Golden Gate Bridge was the exact halfway point between my home and my office. Isn't that cool?). Then, I would drive up highway 101, past Sebastopol (the artist town), and the rest through wine country. It would take me one hour and forty minutes to get to work in the morning and two hours coming back home in the evening, because of heavier traffic, before I reached the Golden Gate Bridge.

Now imagine that I had to think about every little thing I did with the car and the road just to make it to my office in one piece. Imagine my brain using 100% of its capabilities just to get me safely to the office. I bet that by the time I would have reached the office I would have been exhausted. I probably would not be able to do that every morning and evening, and either quit TI or asked my family to move up to Santa Rosa, which we weren't planning to do. Instead, I made this commute for one year and five months (not every day—I worked from home one day a week and travelled quite a bit, which made my commute much shorter, from home to the San Jose International Airport). I enjoyed commuting. And because those habits took such a small part of my brain activity, 95% of it was available for anything else. I bought a digital voice recorder and recorded my thoughts along that 100 to 120 minute drive. I enjoyed the scenery.

***

Using the 80/20 rule, I would say that 20% of the brain is occupied with supporting our habits (even if those represent 80% of our activities), while 80% of the brain is occupied with the special, different, creative, unique things that are *not* habits (even if those represent only 20% of what we do). That part of the brain that deals with the 80% of automatic activities is called the *Basal Ganglia* and is a small, tadpole-shaped, golf ball-sized organ close to the brain stem[23] and to the Hypothalamus, which is responsible to keeping our weight. We will return to the Hypothalamus later in this chapter.

Weight loss and exercise are no fun. If these topics occupied the 80% of the brain that needs to think all the time, we would probably quit losing weight and exercising as a whole, just as I would have quit driving to Santa Rosa. Our goal (and my specific goal in this chapter) is to turn your weight loss (and mine) into a habit. Move it from the 80% to the 20% (the Basal Ganglia) and not spend a second thinking about it.

***

But I don't think I can talk about the theory of habits and the process of creating them without mentioning (and giving credit to) Charles Duhigg, the author of the brilliant book *The Power of Habit*[24].

The process of creating (and maintaining) habits is described by Duhigg as a three-step cycle: a *cue*, a *routine*, and a *reward*. He adds a fourth element (albeit not as a fourth step): the *craving* for the reward that makes us crave the cue. I modified this diagram slightly and described it as a four-step process:

---

[23] The neural network of the basal ganglia as revealed by the study of synaptic connections of identified neurons: A. David Smith and J. Paul Bolam: http://www.mrc.ox.ac.uk/sites/default/files/pdfs/smith1990tins.pdf
[24] Duhigg, Charles, The Power of Habit: Why we do what we do in life and business

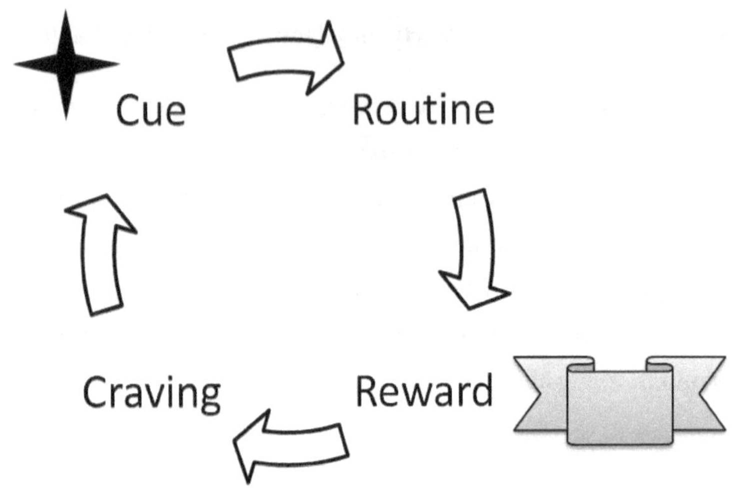

Figure 7: The four steps of the habit loop

First, there is the *cue*. The cue happens regularly and predictably. It invokes the habit *routine*, which, upon completion of it, provides the *reward*. The reward creates the *craving* to feel the cue again to start the process again because, after a while, a consistent and predictable while, our brain will know that the *cue* is followed by the *reward*.

In fact, Duhigg also applied his method to "How to design a New Year's resolution that sticks," specifically applicable to adding the exercise routine to your day[25].

***

It became painfully obvious that the key to a sustainable weight loss for me was to develop new habits. So I decided that I

---

[25] http://charlesduhigg.com/got-a-new-years-resolution-heres-how-to-make-it-stick/

                                                   Yoram Solomon

would lose those 32 pounds over six months, but not faster. That meant approximately five pounds per month. That's sustainable and can become habitual after such a long time of continuous effort. I started in July at approximately 232 pounds and planned to be under 200 pounds by January 1. Six months to lose some 30 pounds—achievable.

However, this could not have been a one-step action. I couldn't be at 232 pounds on December 31st and drop 32 pounds that night to be under 200 pounds the next day. It had to be gradual. At the same time, simply drawing a line between 232 pounds in early July to 200 pounds in January would mean that I needed to track a different number every day, which would be hard to remember. Even assigning a weekly goal is hard to track, as we don't exactly know which week we are on (Did you know that the week of April 10, 2014 is week 15 in the year?). But we certainly know what month we are in, so if I was to lose "only" five pounds per month, I could keep track of my progress. So I decided to set up the following goals:

> For the month of July, I will have to weigh under 228 pounds;
>
> In August, under 222 pounds;
>
> In September, under 216 pounds;
>
> In October, under 210 pounds;
>
> In November, under 205 pounds (now dropping only 5 pounds a month);

Finally, in January and thereafter I will have to weigh under 200 pounds (now dropping the last 5 pounds over *two* months).

You can see that the curve is becoming pretty shallow toward the end, from six pounds per month initially to five pounds over two months eventually, creating a habit of only maintaining my weight after January, neither gaining nor losing any more weight.

This is easy to remember. At any point in time I have known my exact limit. Furthermore, I knew that as I got close to the end of the month, I needed to be closer to next month's weight limit rather than this month's, as there was probably no way I would lose five or six pounds in the last day of the month. I also didn't want to lose that amount in one day because, again, it would not create new diet habits.

Of course, I used an Excel spreadsheet to track my goals and my progress. I drew the "staircase" line of the "official" allowable weight limit, a linear line that connected the points to assure that by the time I get closer to the end of the month I will be closer to next month's weight limit, and finally, a linear line two pounds *under* the previous one, just to assure that I am nowhere near the weight limit. Not losing my RC hobby privileges was just too important.

Every morning I weighed myself, and that was the measurement that mattered. I entered it into the spreadsheet. I compared it to the linear lines. I even inserted "conditional formatting" that changed the color if I was "at risk" of crossing the line in the wrong direction (up). You don't have to do all of this. Knowing (and remembering) the weight limit for this month and next month is enough. Knowing that after the middle of the month you need to be closer to next month's goal than this month's goal is trivial.

A simpler, less "geeky" way of doing this is to print a table that has approximately six months in it (with daily lines). Each line should have the date, the allowed weight for the current month, the "straight line" weight for the day (on a line between the weight limit this month and that of the next month), and then three empty columns to fill your weight in the morning, your weight when you get back home in the afternoon/evening, and your weight at night before you go to bed.

Date	Limit	Line	Morn.	Eve.	Night	
4/1	185	185.0				
4/2	185	184.8				
4/3	185	184.6				
⋮	⋮	⋮	⋮	⋮	⋮	⋮
4/30	185	179.2				
5/1	179	179.0				

The table example above shows that the weight limit for the month of April was 185 lb. If the weight limit for May was 6 lb. lighter (179 lb.), then while 185 lb. is the "official" weight for the month of April, every day I should lose 0.2 lb., and thus on April 2nd I should weigh 184.8 lb. This column is meant to help me not exceed the weight limit on the first day (or few days) of *next* month, if I only observed (and complied with) the current monthly weight limit listed in the second column. The next three columns are empty, and are for *you* to fill in your *actual* weight that you measured in the morning, evening, and night. Finally, it could be useful to leave another column to write comments about weight loss that day, in case something special occurred on a given day. It can help you get to know your body and metabolism better.

***

This book started by explaining that the reason it is so hard for us to lose weight is that the effort required to lose weight is greater than the intrinsic Net Present Value of our long-term health—because we are lazy. Let's harness this laziness to our benefit. Our brains will force us to follow a routine through the creation of habit, if it happens time and time again and the circumstances are the same. The way to make weight loss a habit is to put it into a habitual environment. The best environment for most people (it was for me) is the *morning* routine, as it is so much more prescriptive and cuts across all days of the week compared to the *evening* routine, which can be different every day of the week. Let me take you through my morning routine:

06:00   My wife's alarm clock goes off. I stay in bed and watch TV;

06:30   My own alarm clock goes off. I get out of bed;

06:40   I start my workout on the treadmill, watching YouTube and other videos;

07:00   The TODAY show starts, I watch the headlines, and then continue to watch videos on my iPad;

07:15   I'm done with my workout;

07:15   *Morning weigh-in*, then shower;

07:30   Out of the shower, getting something light to eat;

07:40   Taking Shira to school, and then to the office.

I can get into greater detail than that. I'll tell you that I spend the first minute at a speed of 4 mph on the treadmill at an incline of 1%. Every one minute I increase the incline by 1%, and the speed by 0.1 mph, until I reach 6% incline at a speed of 4.5 mph. I stay on this setting until I reach 2 miles. Then, I go down to 4 mph at 3% incline, and, when I reach 30 minutes (very close to 7:10), I lower to 3 mph and 1%. After about one more minute I'm done.

I know. This sounds very monotonous and unexciting. There will be trainers that will tell you to "spice it up": change your routine, make your routine more interesting. But I propose exactly the opposite: turn your routine into a *habit*, and to do that— everything must stay the same until our lazy brains decide that a shortcut can emerge through exercising this way every morning, and, thus, it should move from the outer layers of our brains to the inner, habit-controlling, *Basal Ganglia*. If you add variety, you might effectively *prevent* your workout routine from becoming a habit. This is also the reason why my evening workout is inconsistent and rare: every evening is different, and it requires a *positive* action to add the workout into my evening routine (which is far from being routine)—not that I don't work out at evenings, but it is rare.

Alex, too, exercises in the morning. He rides his bike for 60 minutes. He does that every morning at 7:15. That's his cue. Like me, he finds it so much easier to turn it into a habit when done during the most routine part of the day.

***

The power of habit can apply to the food you eat as well. I can now understand why some diets recommend only eating one type of food and completely avoiding another (for example, the Atkins Diet that allows you to eat meat but completely prevents you from eating any source of carbohydrates, such as potatoes, bread, or pasta). Part of the rationale behind it is that if you *completely* avoid a certain type of food, then you create a *habit* of avoiding it, to the point where you don't need this food anymore, and therefore don't crave it. Your brain will make that shortcut for you. My path was a little different: I simply ate less, but didn't restrict myself to specific types of food. Maybe this is a way for me to modify my own diet.

***

However, even entering the exercise into my most routine time of the day, the morning, does have its drawbacks. The *weekend* schedule is typically different. The girls don't go to school. I don't go to work. The alarm clock doesn't go off at 6:30AM (and my wife's doesn't go off at 6:00). So I don't work out in the morning on weekends. As a result, I believe that I work out probably half of the weekend days—on average only once every weekend, and typically not during the morning.

The same is true for school breaks. When my wife and daughters sleep late during break, even though I have to go to work and my alarm clock will go off at 6:30, I can't work out. It is simply too noisy and will wake them up. Poor babies. So I don't work out often when school is out.

In both cases I am forced to find another time during the day to work out, even though it is not as routine as the normal, school day, workday morning. However, turning a workout into habit does put pressure on me to do it, anyway.

I don't have this problem when they go to Israel for 3 to 4 weeks during the summer. I am not waking anyone up. In fact, since I already have my iPad on my treadmill, and since Israel is 8 hours ahead of Texas, I use the time to speak with them over Skype, while working out. I hear about everything they have done today and last night, and by the time we're done talking, it is almost time to get off the treadmill!

***

When it was time for my class of Leadership Plano to choose a class project, we almost unanimously chose to launch the first TEDx event in Plano, TEDxPlano[26]. For those of you not familiar with TED Talks, you are missing something important. TED is a non-profit organization committed to bring "ideas worth spreading" to the world, in the form of videos, no longer than 18 minutes each. Some of the world's best speakers and presenters have their own "TED Talk" on www.ted.com. I watch TED Talks all the time. With more than 1,600 videos, top ones with tens of millions of views[27],

---

[26] www.tedxplano.org

[27] At the writing of this book, the top TED video is Ken Robinson's "How Schools Kill Creativity", with more than 27 million views

this is one of my best sources of inspiration. And also something I do when I work out.

So it wasn't a surprise that I was a strong proponent of taking on TEDxPlano as our class project. When you want to hold a local TEDx event, one requirement is that at least 25% of the talks in your event will be pre-recorded TED talks. Thus, one of the tasks we had was to curate videos, which is when I encountered a very interesting (at least to me) talk by Sandra Aamodt[28], called "Why dieting doesn't usually work[29]." At first, this talk contradicted what I wrote here. However, as you think about it at a higher level, you will see that it really doesn't.

She believes that "your brain…has its own sense of what you should weigh, no matter what you consciously believe." She calls this a "set point" and refers to is as a 10-15 pound *range* in which you can make choices to be on the higher or lower end, but that it is much, much harder to stay out of it. Ms. Aamodt attributed this thermostat-like operation to the Hypothalamus, a part of our brains, near the brain stem, and next to the *Basal Ganglia*. According to her, even if you *deliberately* decide to change your weight (either direction), your brain will send strong signals (hunger or fullness) to get back to your set point range, as Figure 8 illustrates.

---

[28] http://www.sandraaamodt.com/
[29]
http://www.ted.com/talks/sandra_aamodt_why_dieting_doesn_t_usually
_work

                                    Yoram Solomon

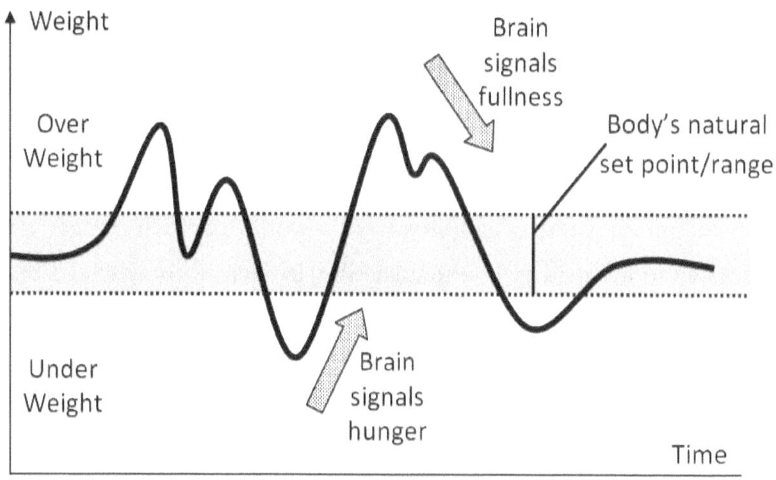

Figure 8: The body's set point

Even though I'm making the case for weight loss here, I agreed with Sandra Aamodt until now. But here is where we disagree. She claimed that "Successful dieting doesn't lower your set point. Even after you kept your weight off for as long as seven years, your brain keeps trying to make you gain it back." She does agree, though, that in light of a long famine, lowering that set point would be a sensible response. She classified eaters into "*intuitive* eaters," who use hunger to control their eating habits, and "*controlled* eaters," who use willpower to control their diet. Those "controlled eaters", according to Aamodt, are more vulnerable to advertising, supersizing, and all-you-can-eat buffets.

She contradicted herself when defining "mindful eating": eat when you are hungry, and stop when you are full. But if our Hypothalamus would force us back to our set point, why do we need to be mindful when we eat? Why not simply rely completely on the Hypothalamus to control eating? After all, if we eat too much, wouldn't the Hypothalamus cause us to feel full, and we would return to the so-called "natural weight"?

The answer comes from a previous part in her talk, when she acknowledged that the set point has increased over time (centuries) with changes in food availability, from a world in which hunger was pervasive to a world of abundance. She, in fact, acknowledged that the set point may change over time.

This, to me, brings an interesting concept from the electrical engineering space. This is the concept of the low-pass filter. The low pass filter is an element that ignores high-speed signal changes and only passes through those changes that are consistent over time. The same can be observed in mechanical engineering in the behavior of *springs*. When you pull a spring, it becomes longer, but as soon as you release it, it will go back to its original size. When you push it, it becomes shorter, but as soon as you release it, it again goes back to its original size. However, if you continue to pull on it over and over again consistently, while it returns to the general length it had before the pull, you will notice that over time that length becomes longer—slightly but longer, as if the spring succumbs to this continuous pull on it, over a long period of time.

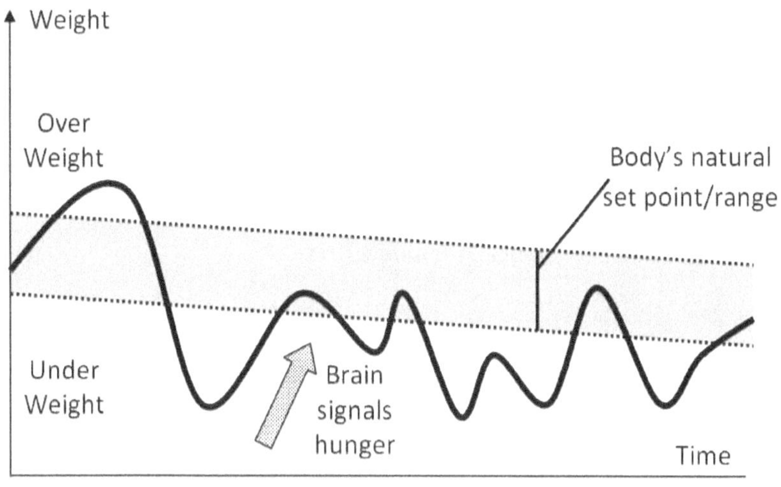

Figure 9: The set point changes slightly over time with continuous effort

Our Hypothalamus may force us back to our natural set point. If we lose weight more than the lower end of the set point range, our brains will instruct us to go back to that set point. If we eat to the point we exceed the high end of the set point range, our brains will instruct us to go back to the set point range. However, if we continue to push weight down through diet, over time—over a *long* period of time, that set point will change, and now the Hypothalamus will "guide" us back to a new set point, as illustrated in Figure 9. Much like we are creating new eating and exercise routine habits that become second nature, our brains adjust to the new weight and will work to maintain and guide us back to it. This is another very good reason to lose weight *gradually* rather than over a short period of time. Let our brains get used to a new reality.

***

But habits also have an amazingly *positive* effect on how hard diet and exercise really are. Just like driving (and any other effort) becomes easier and less stressful the more you do it, as it becomes a habit, so are the efforts associated with diet and exercise. They become easier. You don't have to think about them all the time. But they have to become *habits* first.

Don't try to lose all the weight in one month, as you will not be able to keep it off. Losing it over a longer period of time, more gradually, will create new healthy habits and let you fight your body's inertia and keep that weight off forever.

5.

IT'S A MATTER OF SCALE

I leased my last two cars. When you lease cars, you need to select your annual mileage "allowance" for the lease. That allowance plays a role in determining the residual value of the car when you return it at the end of the lease, and as a result, your monthly payments. If you elect a *high* mileage allowance, you pay more. If you elect a *low* allowance, you pay less. However, when it's time to return the car, if you exceeded that allowance, you have to pay a penalty. So you need to pretty accurately estimate your mileage in the next three years or so. Estimate high and you pay too much during the lease period. Estimate too low and you pay the penalty. When I leased my 2010 car, I estimated 12,000 miles a year. It's a pretty conservative estimate. However, when it was time to return the car after three years, I realized that I drove less than 10,000 miles a year on average. I didn't have to pay a penalty, but I obviously overpaid in the monthly payments. It was probably not too much, but still. So when I leased my 2013 car, I was smarter. I elected a 10,000 mile a year allowance. And that's when things went wrong. Not even three months after I got the car I found myself in the middle of an election to the school board. I was driving all over town, accumulating more miles than I have ever before. After the elections, I felt that I had too many miles, but didn't know exactly how many. Not that the math was so difficult, but I didn't see a reason to calculate it. In early April 2014, just as I started writing this book, I realized that I had more than 18,000 miles on the odometer, when I was supposed to have no more than 15,000. There was no doubt that I was going to return this car with more miles than the allowance, which would have been 30,000 miles by the time I need to turn the car in. I checked the lease agreement and found that I would have to pay 20 cents per mile over the allowance. If I had 3,000 miles over my allowance halfway through the lease, I was going to have 6,000 miles over the allowance by the end of it. Not that paying $1,200 is the end of the world, but I didn't want to pay that. So I've put myself on a "diet." I calculated the number of miles per week I could drive on this car such that by the end of the lease I will have 30,000 (I had less than 12,000 miles left to reach that, over a period of 18 months). I then calculated that I was "allowed" to drive no more than 145 miles per week to meet that goal. Knowing that, I had reset the trip odometer every Monday morning and counted how many miles I drove that week. Every morning, I would compare my wife's and my planned driving dis-tances for the day, and whoever had the shortest trips would take *my* car. I drove 131 miles the first week of this "diet." This increased my weekly allowance (to reach 30,000 miles by the end of the lease term) by just a bit (less than 0.2 miles per week). However, during the fol-lowing weeks I drove 61, 67, 78, and 98 miles. Each week therefore added to the weekly allowance. By the fifth week, my weekly allow-ance was already at 152.6 miles. By the time this book went out to print, my weekly allowance was already above 167 miles, and if I maintain the average weekly mileage I did for the first 18 weeks since I started measuring and tracking it—I would return the car with less than 25,000 miles. Well below my goal.

What does this mean? I couldn't have been on a path to meet the 30,000 mile limit if I hadn't started to measure my miles on a weekly (and daily) basis. You can't be successful if you don't know *when* you are successful, and you won't know that until you have something to *measure.*

***

Many people told me that you should not weigh yourself every day. It can only lead to disappointment and discouragement due to short-term weight gains, even if overall you are losing weight. "Weigh yourself once a week. That's enough," I was told repeatedly. I don't buy that. I weigh myself three times a day. But let me start with explaining why weighing yourself is so important and why it is so important to *this* program. First of all, in my opinion, you cannot improve what you cannot *measure.* In the 1980s there was a management movement around "the Balanced Scorecard[30]." It focused on improving company performance by measuring the *right* parameters, whether financial or otherwise. What you want to measure may be a *trailing* indicator, which means that it will show results only after the actions taken to achieve that result have been in play for a while. Company spending on research and development efforts, for example, will only yield financial results a few years after that spending was made, so your ability to measure the effectiveness of your research and development efforts is delayed.

What about weight loss? Well, we are lucky here because you *can* see the results of your work every day. If you ate too much, it would show even today. If you didn't work out today, it would also show. If you did everything as planned, you will see results. But more than all, *you* have a different body and metabolism than I do.

---

[30] Kaplan, R. S., & Norton, D. P. (1996). The balanced scorecard: Translating strategy into action.

What works for me may not work as well for you, and what doesn't work for me might do wonders for your ability to lose weight, so your ability to measure what does or does not work for you is tied to your own measurements, as frequently as possible. On the other hand, measuring your weight only once a week, or even less frequently than that, will become a trailing indicator, showing the results of your work long after it was expended, preventing you from knowing what works for you and what doesn't.

But there is another reason to weigh yourself every day. If you find out tomorrow that you are two pounds over your desired weight limit, you *can* correct it (eat less, workout more) quickly within a day or two. But if you weigh yourself once a month, and find that you are five (or even ten) pounds overweight, you could get discouraged enough to drop out of the race altogether.

As I told you in the previous chapter, I weigh myself three times a day: once in the morning, once when I get back from work, and once before I go to sleep. These measurements have different purposes. Since I typically weigh the least in the morning, I use this measurement to determine whether I met my goal for the day or not. By the way, cheating is ok. I know, you didn't expect me to say that. I found that my scale shows 0.7 pounds less if I shift my weight to my right foot. Although digital, it's a cheap scale. It doesn't do that on my left foot, so I found that the best results are when I lean on my right. So, I cheat. And it doesn't matter; because once I did it once, the bar is now 0.7 pounds higher (or lower) for my weight loss tomorrow.

Throughout the day I work. I'm somewhat active, some days more than others. I eat. Sometimes I go on business lunches and eat a little more. Some days I just feel like eating more regardless of meetings. When I get back home I weigh myself and know where I stand. I still have a few hours to do something about it.

I will sometimes trade lunch for dinner. When I know there is an event I have to go to where dinner will be served, and I know that I will either not be able to resist eating or will feel uncomfortable being the only person at the table not eating, I will skip lunch (or have a very light one) and have dinner that day. When I get back home from work, I know what kind of dinner I can afford. And then, I weigh myself right before I go to bed. This one really helps me tie together everything I have done in a day—the food I ate; the amount of exercise I had; everything. There is nothing I can do about it anymore, and it tells me exactly what I will weigh in the morning because I know how much I will lose at night. I typically lose some 1.8 to 2 pounds a night. So, if I weighed 204.2 pounds at night, I will likely weigh 202.2 to 202.4 the following morning. It is important for me to weigh myself in the morning anyway because it is the start of a new day. I don't want to guess or calculate how I start each day; I want to know exactly, even if I cheat and shift my weight to my right foot.

***

Buy a digital scale. A $20-40 one would do just fine. You don't need memory or any other fancy feature, but they are accurate. Make sure you get one with tenths pounds. You are not going to lose 5 pounds a day. But you may be 0.3 pounds lighter tomorrow morning than you were this morning. 0.3 pounds may sound like nothing, but if you keep this pace you will lose 100 pounds in a year. That is quite a bit! It's more than what I lost. Although, I didn't plan on losing more than I did. Analog scales (the ones with a needle instead of digits) are not accurate enough and don't give you the granularity of tenths of pounds. This is important. There is also friction in their mechanical mechanism that may cause you to get slightly different results (possibly even a pound off) when you measure several times. Just get a digital scale.

I wear nothing when I weigh myself. I know, I know: too much information. But even if you don't like my free spirit, make sure you wear exactly the *same* clothes (or underwear) every time you weigh yourself. OK, I mean the same type of clothes, not exactly the same ones. You'll be surprised how much clothes weigh, and if you are to weigh yourself with a tenth of a pound accuracy, you need to be able to compare apples to apples. One pair of shoes I own weighs about 1.2 pounds more than another pair. Jeans weigh much more than dress pants, and so on. Now, you are going to start asking yourself: Do I weigh more today because I'm wearing heavier clothes? So, wear the same thing every time you weigh yourself. Or wear nothing. Just be consistent.

Finally, whichever measurement of the day is the one that "counts," keep a log of your progress. You don't have to log all three measurements you took in a day, even though that's what I do and recommend, but make sure you log the one that counts.

***

All diet books focus on "doing the right *thing.*" Each will tell you the *right* things to eat, the *wrong* things to eat, the *right* way to exercise, and the *wrong* way to exercise. Of course, the assumption is that what's good for one person is good for everyone. The idea in this book behind weighing yourself frequently is that rather than just

                                                    Yoram Solomon

"doing the right thing," instead, you should "do the right things that will give you the right *results.*" I am making a few assumptions:

The first is that we are all different. My metabolism is different than yours. What works for me may not work as well for you, and what works for you may not be as effective for me. It might be an issue of different metabolism but might simply be a matter of different schedules and preferences that make certain things impossible for me—or for you.

The second assumption is that you are intelligent enough to figure out what works for you and what doesn't. Measuring your weight three times a day will go a long way to help you figure this out. If you weigh yourself once a month, of even once a week, you will have little opportunity to know what foods worked, what didn't work, and how effective was your exercise routine. But if you do it three times a day, you will very quickly learn exactly what worked and what didn't. You will even find out the *interactions* between different types a food, interaction between eating and exercising, doing things at different times during the day, etc. I don't think you should write these things down or use an app that will help you track those. You will figure it out pretty quickly.

My third and final assumption is (pay careful attention to this one) that once you know what works and what doesn't, you will do more of the things that work and less of the things that don't. Talk about stating the obvious.

As I read this part to my wife, she made a good point: "What you are saying sounds like a pure case of 'the end justifies the means,' and this is not true. You can have the same calorie intake by starving yourself and allowing only small portions of very unhealthy food (her example was chocolate), which should not be compared to eating healthy food with the same caloric value." So let me qualify my point. You should make healthy choices. The goal of this book is not to tell you *what* those healthy choices are. As I stated in the beginning, I believe that you are intelligent enough to tell good nutrition from bad, and if not, you know where to find this information. The point I was making is simply that the *results* should be driving you.

We already established that your body is different than mine; your metabolism is different than mine, and what works for me might not work for you. This brings us back to one of the reasons I mentioned weighing yourself frequently is so important: you get to know your own body. If my weight in the morning when I get out of bed is 200 pounds, then after I burn 350 calories on the treadmill I'm typically 0.3 to 0.4 pounds less. This is a good time to mention that I actually weigh myself *before* I work out in the morning and *after* the workout. It really doesn't take much effort to squeeze two weigh-ins in the morning, when I'm already wearing exactly the same things. The slight weight loss (0.3 to 0.4 pounds, and sometimes more if I work out longer or harder) serves another purpose: it is my immediate gratification, or a mini-reward required for the habit cycle to be complete. I can see the immediate impact of my routine. When I get home from work in the evening, assuming I had a normal lunch and had a normal physical activity level, my weight would typically be around 202 to 205 pounds. If I don't eat anything else that evening, I will weigh about 2 pounds less by the time I go to bed, and another 2 pounds less over the course of the night (my metabolism works at night as well!). You need to find your own cycle. As time goes by you will get to know it well and be able to, like me, know what your weight will be *before* you get on the scale within 0.2 to 0.3 pounds. The early evening weigh-in tells me what I need to do during the rest of the evening. If I weighed about 202, I can have a reasonable dinner. If my weight is close to 205, I shouldn't eat anything and should squeeze in another workout session on the treadmill. If I weigh close to 204, I should really only get a very light snack, or nothing at all, or a light dinner with a workout. And then I will get up in the morning still at 200.

Because this is so important and key to the success of this diet, I have to repeat it again. Your weight loss success is not through focusing on doing the right *things* (food and exercise), but on the right things that give you the right *results* (weight) and the way to find what gives *you* the right results. You need to weigh yourself three times a day.

***

It is now time to see how the survey I conducted addresses this theory. To do that, I asked myself two questions. The first question was, "What is the effect of the *frequency* in which the participants weighed themselves on how much weight they were able to lose?" Of the 222 participants, 63 weighed themselves at least once a day ("high frequency") and 159 weighed themselves once a week, once a month, or even less frequently than that. 49% of those who weighed themselves frequently lost 10 lb. or less, while 51% lost 20 lb. or more (a few even lost more than 100 lb.). However, of the 159 participants who weighed themselves less frequently, 60% lost 10 lb. or less, while 40% lost 20 lb. or more. This means that:

If you weigh yourself once or more a day, you have 11% high-er probability to lose a significant amount of weight, compared to if you weigh yourself less frequently than that.

The second question I wondered about was this: "What is the effect of the *frequency* of in which participants weighed themselves on their ability to *keep the weight they lost off* for a prolonged period of time?" Here, I first filtered the participants and only analyzed those who have lost at least 10 lb., at least 3 months before answering the survey. A total of 117 participants qualified for this analysis. Of those who weighed themselves less frequently, 49% kept most of the weight off, while 51% gained most (if not all, or even more than they lost) back. However, of those who weighed themselves at least once a day, 71% kept most (if not all) of the weight off, while only 29% gained most (if not all, or more) back. This is even a more powerful finding:

If you weigh yourself once or more a day, you have 22% high-er probability to keep most of the weight you lost off, compared to if you weigh yourself less frequently than that.

Yoram Solomon

You need to weigh yourself three times a day. This way you can quickly react to a temporary weight gain, but also you get to know your body and metabolism, and know what works for you and what doesn't. Don't just do "the right things," do the right things that give you "the right results."

6.

THE CARROT AND THE STICK

We have established that intrinsic-internal motivation (health, looks, longevity), *because* it is so far in the future, is going to be less effective once it is discounted and the little motivation resulting from its Net Present Value is simply not enough to motivate us to take on the hard effort of diet and exercise.

If there is no strong motivation, you will always be able to rationalize *not* working out or eating slightly *more.* Have you ever made the following excuses?

1. My muscles hurt; I can't work out today;

2. I'm too tired;

3. I'll only eat this today, and tomorrow start my diet;

We don't need much to avoid the effort associated with weight loss because there is no strong motivation.

We then have to resort to extrinsic-external motivators, those that have *nothing* to do with the direct benefits of weight loss (looks, health, longevity) but, rather, other things that we care about, even if they are completely unrelated to weight loss.

However, in order for an external-extrinsic motivator to be effective it has to have a *reward that is contingent upon meeting my weight loss goals.* And that is the key. This relationship between the diet and the reward, albeit not a natural one (like that between the diet and my health), has to be *strong.* I get the reward *only* if I meet my daily diet goals. Only then this reward meets the criteria of being the one required for the creation of the habit cycle described by Duhigg. The extrinsic-external motivator therefore needs to be the following:

1. It has to be something that is *important* to you. Something that makes life fun. For example, for me it is my RC hobby. I love it. I spent a lot of time and effort on it. If somehow you told me that if I don't put the effort required to meet my weight loss goals I will not be able to practice this hobby, I will do it. It is *that* important to me. The value of this hobby is more than the "pain" associated with the weight loss effort. Obviously the immediate benefit from this hobby is more important to me than the (discounted) Net Present Value of the direct weight loss benefits, or I wouldn't need this as a motivator at all. The motivator could be to drive your new car (when your old car is still around). Again, you need to find out what meets this criterion for *you.* Don't try what works for me or anyone else.

2. It has to be something that will not *hurt* you or others if you can't do it (because you didn't meet your daily goal): you (and others) can live without it. I can live without my hobby. Nobody will be hurt if I don't get to practice it. Granted, I might become grumpy at home (and work) and not pleasant to be around, but it will not really *hurt* me or anyone else. If, for example, I would determine that I can't go to work on days when I didn't meet my goals, this could hurt my com-

                                   Yoram Solomon

pany that will not get the outcome of my work, and my family, as they will not benefit from my income. If I decided that I will not teach the Junior Achievement class that I taught every Friday if I didn't meet my goal, the kids at Renner Middle School will suffer. It has to be something that I (and the rest of the world) can live *without,* albeit I wouldn't have fun—of some sort. It still has to be important enough to be a strong enough motivator.

3. It has to be something that you care about *every day,* not just occasionally. This works with weighing yourself every day. Just like I need to weigh every day to make sure that my weight doesn't get out of hand to the point I cannot recover from it, I need the motivator to be something I exercise every day. If, for example, I chose something that I only do on weekends (sail my boat in the lake), then I might lose track of my weight-loss effort and only at the weekend find out whether I can sail or not, and by then it would be too late. I do something with my RC hobby *every day*—whether it's buying parts, tools, materials, (or even whole planes), building something, or flying. I will miss it a lot if I had to go a day without it. Sure, there are days in which I don't do anything with my hobby because I'm too busy with something else, but generally I do something every day.

4. It has to be something that already requires significant investment of effort, time, and money. In other words, you already have a vested interest in *continuing* it. For example (more in the next chapter), let's say that I have a brand new luxury (or sport) car, while I still have the older, cheaper

"clunker" (that still runs) available. I will allow myself to drive the new car only on days I meet my goals. I can promise you that I will not let myself drive the clunker and write off the purchase of the luxury or sport (or sport-luxury) car. I have already invested a lot of time, effort, and money in my RC hobby. I spent more than 500 building hours on one of the planes I built, for example. There is no way that I will accept that I cannot lose weight and, therefore, will never be able to complete that plane or fly it. Still, nobody will really get *hurt* if I didn't.

5. Feel free to allow yourself on bad days (days in which you didn't meet your daily goals and thus was prevented from the extrinsic motivating reward) to increase the importance of the motivator to you. I am allowed to communicate over the Internet forums associated with my RC hobby on those bad days. I can go to my flying field/club and see what the *others* are doing even on days in which I didn't meet my weight loss goals. Those only *increase* the value of the motivator for me. I see others fly, and I hear about others who build and fly, yet stupid me, I can't do anything today because I didn't meet my goals today. I'll make sure I meet it tomorrow.

When the consequences are *clear* (and unrelated to long-term health or a promise you made to yourself with no enforcement mechanism) and of *significance* to you, you will not make excuses to why you cannot meet your goals today. You are not going to be too tired. You will not eat just that one dessert that you know will take you over the limit. You will simply do what you have to do to meet your goals.

***

This extrinsic motivator is important to get us to overcome the effort associated with eating less and exercising more. It acts as the reward required for Duhigg's habit creation cycle. Specifically, in the case of exercise, there can be another reward: the weight measured right *after* the workout. As you weigh yourself right after workout and find that you lost some weight (even if it is less than half a pound), it becomes an immediate reward to complete the habit creation cycle albeit a smaller reward than that associated with your ability to conduct whatever it is you made contingent upon meeting your weight goal. It is more immediate in most cases, and, thus, it adds to the overall effectiveness of the cue-routine-reward cycle.

***

But so far we only discussed *what* will be a strong enough motivator, albeit extrinsic-external, but not the *enforcement* mechanism of it. What would make the *link* between the effort (eat less, exercise more) and reward (practice your hobby) *unbreakable*? In other words, who said that I cannot work on my hobby on a day in which I didn't meet my weight-loss goals? Read the next chapter.

The motivation to go through the effort of weight loss cannot come from your long-term health. It has to be completely external, daily, and must be really important to you.

7

GIVE THE KEYS TO SOMEONE ELSE

The problem starts with the fact that the low Net Present Value of the intrinsic-natural motivator (your long-term health) is not enough, and the extrinsic motivator we need to use is not naturally linked to the weight loss effort, and, therefore, this weak link can easily be broken—by *you*.

In the previous chapter you determined *what* the extrinsic motivator is and what the daily consequences for not meeting your goals should be. But what will keep you *honest*? What will make this link unbreakable? Again, this will be different for *you* than it is for me or everyone else. This is the "enforcement" part of the diet. We tend to cut corners. I was only 0.3 pounds above my weight limit for the day, but I really needed to go flying today with my buddies. I promised them! This is no longer about me. This is about *them*! Or, "Let's keep things in proportion here, after all we are doing this for my own health, and right now what will make me healthy is to go flying my airplanes!"

You can have this conversation with yourself. God knows I had these conversations with myself—many times. And if it were purely up to me, I would have lost this debate and go do what I wanted to do even though I didn't meet my goals. This starts a slippery slope of not meeting goals. What happens tomorrow? Where is the line? Is it at 0.3 pounds? Is it at one pound? Two? Ten? You see where this is going.

The best way to fight this is to not cut corners. Easier said than done, but this means it cannot be up to *me* anymore, as I'm simply not strong enough. The best way to keep "objective enforcement" (and the unnatural link between the extrinsic motivator and the required action) in place is to *give someone else the keys.*

***

In a study conducted by Dan Ariely at MIT in 2002[31], 99 executive students were split into two groups. One group was given the dates in which to submit three papers during class. The second group was allowed to *choose* and declare (and commit) to the dates by which they will submit their own papers. There were *penalties* for missing the submission deadlines and *bonuses* for beating those. The results showed that students who *chose* deadlines that were more restrictive with those dates than they had to. Only 27% of the students chose to submit their papers at the last day of class, which was clearly a viable option. They instead chose to commit to submitting them earlier. When left to our own devices, we will impose *harder* restrictions on ourselves than necessary. Furthermore, the result of this study showed that the *performance* (here: a grade) of the student group with *externally* imposed deadlines was *better* than the performance of the students with the self-imposed deadlines. A second study was conducted which included papers to proofread (with "planted" errors to catch). Again, one group was given externally imposed weekly deadlines, while the other group was free to choose

---

31 Dan Ariely and Klaus Wertenbroch (2002), "Procrastination, Deadlines, and Performance: Self-control by Precommitment." Psychological Science, Vol. 13, No. 3: 219-224
(http://dl1.cuni.cz/pluginfile.php/95343/mod_resource/content/0/Ariely_2002_procrastination.pdf)

                                    Yoram Solomon

their own deadlines and committed to them. Again, there were penalties for missing deadlines, and performance (number of errors caught) was measured. And, once again, the performance of the group with *externally* imposed deadlines was significantly *better* than those of the group with self-imposed deadlines (by close to 30%), and delays in submission we much shorter for the group with externally imposed deadlines compared to those with self-imposed deadlines (by close to 30%). We meet externally imposed restrictions, deadlines, and goals better than we meet those we impose on ourselves. Give the keys to someone else.

***

One day I met Matthew for coffee. Matthew has been my friend for twelve years now. He used to drive a Porsche. I asked him about the car and he said that he no longer owned it.

"So, what do you drive now?"

"My wife's old Acura."

OK, at this point I need to mention that I'm also an investor in his startup company, so that didn't make me feel so confident about his company and my investment anymore.

"Why?"

"I'm waiting for my custom order of a Mercedes E-Class to arrive from Germany."

Now I felt much better. He obviously felt good enough about the prospects of his company (and my investment, did I mention this already?) to order this car.

Then he noted that I lost significant weight. I acknowledged losing over thirty pounds, but that happened more than a year ago. I have maintained it for more than a year now.

"How did you do it?" the obvious question. "I want to lose weight as well!"

So, I described the process and the short-term/long-term extrinsic motivation theory behind it.

"How can this apply to me?"

I thought for a second and asked: "Can you keep your wife's old Acura longer?"

"Sure, but why? I wouldn't want to drive it once the Mercedes arrives, though!"

"Exactly! Every day you will be over the allowed weight limit for the month, you will have to drive the old Acura, and every day you are at or below that limit, you can drive the Mercedes!"

"But how can I make sure I don't give myself a break and drive the Mercedes even if I'm over the weight limit?"

"*Give the keys to your wife* or, better yet, to your children. Your wife is more likely to let you 'cut corners' than your children." She may know how hard it is to lose weight (to be clear, I'm not saying or implying that Matthew's wife has, needs to, or ever needed to lose weight. I'm simply stating that adults have a better understanding for how hard it is to cut corners. And no, I'm not saying she cuts corners, either.). That was close…

This is just one example of what *you* can do to find an extrinsic motivator that is important on a daily basis as well as a *gatekeeper* who will prevent you from "breaking the law," thus making the unnatural link unbreakable.

What worked for me is that I promised my *daughters* that I would not buy, build, or fly airplanes if my weight was above the allowed weight limit for the day/month. It's not that they would physically prevent me from doing all those things. They didn't keep a lock on my Internet connection to make sure I didn't buy anything or keep my tools to prevent me from building or keep my car keys to prevent me from going to fly. It wasn't like that at all. They didn't even keep track over my weight or asked me every day if I was "within my limits." So if I violated my rules, I could get away with it and they wouldn't know. But I didn't. I can't lie to my daughters, and I don't ever want to give them a bad example. So, if they had asked me if I was within my limits and I wasn't, I couldn't tell them that I was. To me there is no "white lie" here. It's pretty cut-and-dry. And if I was above my allowed weight limit and, yet, violated my rules and did buy, build, or fly that day, I would have to admit that I violated the rule, thus, showing them a bad example. To me, being a bad example to my daughters is the last thing I want to do. I don't want to portrait myself as a saint or a perfect father, which I'm not, but to me giving my daughters a bad example when their personality is still developing is unacceptable. When they look up to me as a role model, I do not want them to see me as someone who breaks promises. Shira was stricter with me than her sister. I once got slightly above my weight limit for the day and really needed to fly that day. Shira wouldn't let me. She couldn't listen to reason. I appealed the best way I could, but she simply didn't let me cut that corner. She did her job the best way she could, with no bias, prejudice, or flexibility. Why would this not work with my wife? Because her personality is already developed, and I'm not as worried about giving her a bad example. I don't need to worry about her looking up to every mistake I make.

Maybe this doesn't work for you. If not, it doesn't make you a bad person. It's just that *this* enforcement mechanism doesn't work effectively enough for you, and you need something stronger. Consider actually giving someone something that prevents you from doing what you want to do. That person can only give it to you if you are within your limits. If you are not certain that you will always tell the truth (considering the consequences), have that person *verify* your compliance. You will need to be creative here. Remember that dieting is hard. You need strong motivation. Intrinsic motivation doesn't work, and the extrinsic motivation doesn't have a natural link to weight loss efforts. Cutting corners is very tempting, so the enforcement mechanism would need to be strong and objective. It should not be easy to let you cut corners.

I'm not perfect. Throughout 6 months of weight loss I had 12 "bad days" in which my weight was above the allowed limit. In those days, I did not buy, build, or fly. I didn't need someone to actually hold the keys. But what if an exception is really, really needed? For example, our RC club in Aubrey, Texas, holds an annual "Warbirds over Texas" event each June, which attracts flyers from all around the state of Texas and beyond. This event is three days long, and the second day is the best one. What if my weight was above the allowed limit exactly that day? What if I planned to go flying with friends, or what if I promised to teach someone to fly and couldn't do it because of my "deal with the devil?"

                                                      Yoram Solomon

Well, there are two ways around that. One, and the simplest to enforce, is: don't slip! If this is important to you, make double sure that you will not exceed your weight on that day. Maybe you need to build a buffer of a few extra pounds before that day, so that even if you happen to eat too much the day before, you will still not be in violation.

Another thing that worked for me was *coupons*. Yes, coupons. I had Shira (my younger daughter) give me one coupon (of course, I can give myself the coupon, but she really wanted to do it, and was great in creating and enforcing them. She had expiration dates on the coupons) for a "Free Get out of Jail" day. I had one coupon in a year. For one day, if everything stacked against me and I didn't meet my dietary restrictions, I could still buy, build, and fly, using the coupon. But I treasured that coupon. I did everything in my power to not use it. In fact, the first time such a coupon was issued I ended up working extra hard to make sure I didn't use it. The *existence* of the coupon was an extra motivation by itself. As long as the rules are very clear, a rare exception, a well-defined, limited and bound exception could be allowed.

***

Another small example of "giving the key to someone else" is how Alex exercises. Unlike me, he doesn't find working out *inside* the house interesting enough. He rides his bike *outside* every morning. He rides for 60 minutes. However, he rides 30 minutes in *one direction* and then rides back. Riding it some 6 miles one way kind of doesn't leave you with many alternatives to whether you ride the remaining 30 minutes or not.

***

The "give the keys to someone else" concept complements the external motivator as the *enforcement* mechanism. The external motivator will not be effective without a strong enforcement mechanism. The effectiveness of the enforcement mechanism depends on the answer to one question: what are the consequences *to me* of "overriding" the enforcement mechanism? It is important to distinguish between the *reward* for achieving my daily goal (or the penalty for missing it), that was discussed in the previous chapter, and the consequence of disconnecting the unnatural link between achieving the goal and getting the reward. I am talking about the latter here: the consequences of *disconnecting the link* between missing the goal and the punishment (lack of reward) I should experience. The effectiveness of that extrinsic motivator could depend on several things (among other possible):

1. *Who* is in control of the reward associated with the external motivator? Is it someone with authority over me? There are people I am afraid of. My pastor, my rabbi, my boss, or others cause me to think twice before I break my promises *to them.* I would include my daughters too, but not because I'm afraid of them, but rather because I don't want to be bad example. And that's pretty powerful for *me.* The control can be as simple as a lock. I can't reason with a lock. People I respect a great deal have this effect on me. Any sort of person I don't want to let down motivates me to choose wisely.

2. How easy is it to *override* the enforcement mechanism? The enforcement mechanism could be, possibly, technological. Let's assume that my scale had a compartment in it for my brand new car keys (the car is new, not the keys). Let's fur-

                                    Yoram Solomon

ther assume that if I didn't deposit the keys in the compartment at night, an alarm would sound. The scale will be programmed with my allowed weight limit program and will only open if my weight was lower than the weight limit for the day. Finally, let's assume that the scale can recognize me through some biosensor and know that I'm not cheating. There will be no way to override the enforcement mechanism. This could also occur through giving someone else the ability to change the password to my computer, preventing me access unless I proved that I met my daily goals. It should be pretty cut-and-dry and should not be easily overridden.

3.   What are the *consequences* to me if I override the enforcement mechanism? In the case of Dan Ariely's MIT experiment, I will get a lower score. Or I will get paid less for translating papers with grammatical mistakes. Not such a big deal. However, I consider the consequence of being a poor example to my daughter to be significant. Again, it is important to emphasize that this part talked about the consequences of violating the *link* between the extrinsic motivator and the weight loss effort—not the motivator itself.

4.   How *reliable* is the person controlling my enforcement mechanism in keeping me honest? This, again, is where my daughters (especially Shira), are more strict than my wife. She knows how hard it is for adults to lose weight. She is much more understanding of what I'm going through, and therefore she is much more probable to let me override the

mechanism than my daughters are. They never had to lose weight. They don't understand what I'm going through. And that's what makes them perfect.

*⁎⁎

When Don got out of his car he looked different. It was the same Saab convertible I knew for many years, but I wasn't 100% certain that it was the same Don who got out of that car. I couldn't help it, and when he came closer I asked "Where is the rest of you?" Not that Don was ever a "heavyweight" or looked overweight, but the person who met me for lunch that day was thinner—much thinner. I knew Don for about ten years, ever since we both served on the board of the local chapter of the Association for Strategic Planning. Don is a successful executive recruiter with his own firm. We stayed in touch over the years, and about a month ago he sent me a somewhat cryptic email asking me what do I do to cheer myself up? I replied with quite a lot of detail, and it was mostly around my RC hobby. That hobby does take my mind away from other worries and stress. But when I wondered why he would ask me such a question, I reached only one possible conclusion: he must be writing a book. So at the end of my reply to his inquiry I suggested we meet for lunch to discuss his upcoming book. We hadn't met in about three years, so we were long overdue. But when he got out of his car I realized we were not going to talk about his book. We were going to talk about his weight loss. Sure enough, he is writing a book (with a partner) with ideas how to cheer oneself up. But given what Don looks like today, the conversation naturally quickly shifted to his weight loss. Don weighed approximately 230 pounds the last time I saw him, some three years ago, just like me. He was not obese, but did feel the weight. The thought of losing weight has been brewing in his head

                                   Yoram Solomon

for a while, but one morning he woke up and something *snapped.* He was done *thinking* about it, and he was about to *execute.* He didn't like what he looked like, and he didn't like how he felt.

Over the next two and a half years Don lost 70 pounds, and he now weighs 160. He shed 30 percent of his body weight. The interesting thing, though, is that he didn't change his *eating* habits much. Don was not very particular in what he had for lunch that day with me. He didn't avoid anything specific. We just had a good lunch that we both enjoyed. We enjoyed the company and the conversation more than the food (not that the food was bad—on the contrary!), which is an important factor in not eating too much. I can't tell you how many events I went to and how much time I spent enjoying people and conversations; I often forgot to eat.

There is no trick to it; in order to lose weight you need to eat less, exercise more, or better yet, do both. Don didn't eat less, not *much* less anyway. But he exercised more. Don decided to work out in a gym. The gym was on his way to work, so the *friction* associated with going to the gym was minimal. He scheduled two sessions during the week, always the first thing Monday morning before the workweek begun and the last thing Friday afternoon after the workweek was over. This allowed the workout to become a routine: a habit. But he needed to make sure that he goes through with this routine, so Don hired a personal trainer. He is currently working with his *third* trainer. One of the trainers would sometimes not show up on time to the training session. Don is a very punctual professional and couldn't stand that. In fact, we both showed up to our lunch meeting two minutes ahead of time. You could count on Don to be there on time, and he demanded that from the trainer. After all, for the exercise routine to become a habit, it has to occur at a very *pre-*

dictable time, in response to a *cue.* Here, the cue was the *time* itself. The appointments with the trainer are standing appointments. While they can be cancelled, Don's understanding with the trainer is that cancellation should happen no less than three weeks in advance. Unless travel is involved, those appointments will typically not be cancelled. Canceling the appointment less than three weeks in advance could cost Don money, but I don't think that money was the issue, as Don's high level of trustworthiness and integrity will not allow him to cancel an appointment less than three weeks in advance, denying the trainer the opportunity to book an appointment with another client for the same time slot. Don will also not simply *miss* an appointment, even if he knows that he still has to pay his trainer. Don will never do that. And hence *he gave the keys to someone else.* If Don would have decided to work out by himself, without a trainer, he might not have persisted. If he did not care as much about his trainer and would cancel his sessions without (or with little) notice, he would not have been as successful. If his appointments would not take place at very specific times in the week, a habit would not have been formed.

I should add that Don actually works out two more times during the week without a trainer: Wednesdays and Saturdays. But it is the Monday and Friday sessions that "keep him honest." Don insisted that his 70-pound weight loss was purely due to the exercise routine and not his nutrition, but when I asked him what his target weight was, he said that it was 160 pounds, which he reached. When I asked him how he *leveled off* his weight loss, he told me that he started watching less what he ate. So my conclusion is that he *did* watch what he ate *some* but didn't go on a hunger strike. It was the exercise routine that accounted for the bulk of his weight loss. He

                                      Yoram Solomon

told me what he did in every workout session, and some of it included things that I only did during my basic military training—not at our age. But this goes to show that there is no one single way to lose weight. What Don needed was the motivation (in his case, he "snapped" one day), the weight loss routine (in his case, the exercise sessions) that had all the ingredients to make it a habit, and giving the keys to someone else (in his case, his trainer and high sense of integrity). While Don lost 70 pounds, he did it over a two-and-a-half-year period, which translates to less than 2.5 pounds a month. This is a rate that can be relatively easily maintained for a long period of time (enough for it to become a habit) and easy to level off from.

I remain optimistic about Don's ability to maintain his new physique, especially since he had been successful at it for almost three years now. However, it is still too early to tell, as only a few months have passed since he reached his goal. I can't wait to see Don again in another two or three years to learn how he maintained his results.

***

I wanted to finish with a statement from Sandra Aamodt's TED talk, which justifies the "give the keys to someone else" approach: "any strategy that relies on its consistent application is pretty much guaranteed to eventually fail you when your attention moves on to something else." And, in order to make sure that your attention never moves to something else, make sure your motivator is important to you, has consequences (or rewards) every day, and that someone else is in charge of the unnatural link between the motivator and the weight loss effort.

A final instance of "give the keys to someone else" for me is the writing (and mainly publishing) of this book. After all, once I put myself out there, I can imagine people I know asking me how much do I weigh? I can't afford to gain weight. It's out of my hands because of the consequences. It's now in your hands.

The link between the extrinsic motivator and weight loss effort is not a natural one. It is man-made, and you are not to be trusted to keep it. You will cut corners. You have to have someone else hold the keys to your extrinsic rewards or consequences.

8.

AND NOW, FOR THE REST OF YOUR LIFE

As evidenced from my Colt 1911 "experiment," reaching your goal and then letting go doesn't work and has little value. You may start buying clothes that are two (or more) sizes smaller, just to find that two-three months later you don't fit in them anymore. All the health results that your doctor and you raved about will make room for the same old conversations with your doctor:

"You need to lose weight."

"I know."

In fact, you would probably be even more frustrated, and possibly more disappointed with yourself, and when you are disappointed, you eat.

In order to transition into the rest of your life, you need to do several things. First, your weight loss plan should stretch over a long period of time such that you will develop new *habits*. Can you lose 30 pounds in one month? Of course you can. But would it create new habits? It won't. What worked for me was a 6-month period. I'm not sure if any research was ever done to define how long does it take to develop certain habits, but at this point I would recommend 6 months. In my research, of those who lost a significant amount of weight (at least 20 pounds) over a period of 3 months or less, 53% managed to keep at least half of the weight they lost off (47% gained it all or more back), while of those who lost the weight over a period of 6 months or more, 65% managed to keep at least half of the weight they lost off (only 35% gained it all, or even more back). In other words:

> *You are 12% more likely to keep most of the weight you lost off if you lost it over a period of 6 months or longer than if you lost it over a shorter period of time.*

12% better likelihood might not sound like a lot. However, 12% due to losing it over a longer period of time, plus 22% due to weighing yourself at least once a day, plus anything from this book that you will practice—these things add up. Anything that will increase your probability for success is worth doing.

Second, the transition into a "flat line" (simply keeping your weight, rather than losing more) should be a *gradual* one. I had to lose 30 pounds. I decided to lose them over 6 months. That means 5 pounds a month. Losing 5 pounds a month are not the same as *maintaining* your weight. This means that on January 1st I had to transition from losing 5 pounds a month to "maintenance" mode. If I continued the same habits I've been adopting for the last 6 months, I would continue and lose 5 pounds a month. If, on the other hand, I would *relax* some of those habits, I would also risk starting to gain the weight back again. The approach should be to determine the weight limits as a line that becomes less and less steep. Bottom line: I would like you to only lose 1 to 2 pounds in the last month. Make it a curve that is manageable. Don't try to lose too much in the first month. For example, my curve (6, 6, 6, 6, 5, 3, 2) allowed me to "level off" and keep my new weight without overcompensating in the first month after I reached my goal. Trying to do (11, 8, 5, 3, 2, 1) would give you a better curve in the end but is somewhat steep at the beginning. Losing 11 pounds in one month requires much more effort than losing 5 or 6. So, try and do something in between. How about (7, 6, 6, 5, 4, 2)? Losing 7 pounds in the first month is not too bad, and losing only 2 pounds in the last month would better prepare you to maintain your weight afterwards. I'm not going to give you a formula. Just use your judgment.

Third, you need to continue and weigh yourself three times a day for the rest of your life. Sounds hard? It really isn't. You already got used to doing it over six months now, so it's not such a terrible burden. However, it is very important to make sure that you do not let yourself go and gain what you lost back simply because you were asleep on your watch—especially if you consider "killing the deal" (see next). I still weight myself three times a day, almost two years after achieving my goal.

Finally, you may decide to "kill the deal" as long as you are maintaining your weight and not gaining any, but in that case give yourself a line. If your target weight is 160 pounds, you will not have to stop what you were enjoying on any day that you were above 160. In my case, I wanted to stay under 200 pounds. When I reached 200 pounds, my physician actually told me to stop losing weight and to simply maintain 200. I figured that I already developed the right habits, so while I continued to weigh myself every day, I allowed myself to go slightly over and then go back to normal, within reason. However, in December 2013 I was 5 pounds over. It is important to draw this line and recognize when you crossed it. At that point I wrote the following email to my daughters:

I didn't manage to keep my weight down. I'm more than 5 pounds over. So, I need to go back to my extrinsic motivation method: I will not buy, build, or fly RC airplanes until I get under 200 lb. again. Please keep me honest on this.

Dad.

So I got back on "the deal": no buying, building, or flying RC airplanes until I reached 200. Once I reached 200 again, I could continue to live without that restriction, but whenever I get up in the morning and find that my weight is over 205, I'm back on the daily restriction. As of the writing of this book, I haven't been back to 205. When I get closer, I start watching myself more than before, but I can continue my hobby as long as I like and practice the *other* hobby as well. But that's a story for another book.

***

In a research paper published at Duke University in 2006[32], researchers claimed that 45% of our daily actions are the result of habits and 55% are not. Some activities can be categorized as both. Driving to work, for example, is a habit, whereas driving on a trip over the weekend is not. We protect our *habitual* activities from change and, thus, those are the hardest ones to modify. Even when people want to change a habit for all the right reasons, they are likely

---

[32] Bas Verplanken and Wendy Wood (2006). Interventions to Break and Create Consumer Habits. Journal of Public Policy & Marketing, 25(1): http://dornsife.usc.edu/assets/sites/208/docs/Verplanken.Wood.2006.pdf

                                    Yoram Solomon

to continue with "the old habits" because the environment that cues them hasn't changed.

The researchers claimed that changing those environmental cues is key to changing habits. However, I will not encourage moving to a new home or getting a divorce for the sole purpose of losing weight. If you hate your job, or can't get along with your spouse, that's a different story. But if you are happy, don't leave them to lose weight.

The researchers further proposed that policy (as in *laws*) changes could affect the environment and, thus, habits, but we will not suggest the government should legislate weight loss. However, if we look carefully at policies, they are made of *rules* and *enforcement*. Consider the daily/monthly weight limits as the *rules*, and the "give the keys to someone else" the *enforcement* mechanism. This is how I propose to change old habits in this book.

Finally, the researchers suggested continuing and reinforcing the environment that was a trigger to the motivation for changing habits. As old habits die, new habits emerge, and maintaining the environment that allowed the new habits to be created becomes essential for their survival. I told you the story of the 1911 pistol milestone. It didn't create new *habits* because it was over a very short period of time, in which old habits didn't die, and new habits were not born. But even if it would have taken me a year to lose that weight, the new nutrition and exercise habits are still fragile after I reached my goal. So, unless I maintain the environment that allowed them to emerge, I will most likely go back to my old habits. You need to continue with the policy (the weight limit, the consequences for not meeting it, and the enforcement mechanism that is maintained by another person and is as out of your control as possible) for longer, possibly *much* longer, and maybe for the rest of your life. You already know it's worth it, and after a while, it doesn't seem as hard as it was initially.

***

You also need to make sure that the source of extrinsic motivation for you continues to be effective, especially over the long-term. Our lives change. Hobbies change. Priorities change. In 2013, for example, I found myself running a campaign for the Plano school board. That took a lot of my time, and didn't leave much for the hobby anyway. So, if I know I can't do anything with my hobby anyway, what's to keep me on my diet? For one, the question is: how strong are the habits I had already developed? They might be strong enough. However, if they are still weak and fragile, and your motivation has changed, adapt!

In 2013, I also took on another hobby. I started practicing for high-power rifle competitive shooting. It was easy for me to drop my involvement in the RC hobby whenever I was over the weight limit and focus on the other hobby. Very quickly I realized that I was doing that, and added the new hobby "under the contract." Now I couldn't do anything with any of the two hobbies while I'm above the weight limit. Granted, my community involvement that resulted from the 2013 campaign started taking a larger part of my life, but I still had time for my hobbies, and I needed those hobbies to keep my sanity. So the contract I made kept the diet going, and my weight is still at (or close to) 200 pounds.

***

Yoram Solomon

Finally, the weight loss itself can help in reinforcing the benefit. Looking better, feeling better, and getting positive feedback (How does it feel when you see someone you haven't seen in a while, and the first statement/question out of their mouth is: "you lost weight"?) are all helping reinforce the benefit and, thus, the new routine.

***

Hopefully I convinced you that the method described in this book, which clearly worked for *me*, may work for *you*, and is within your abilities. But is it? Is there the right and wrong time to start the diet? I never thought about the possibility that this could be something feasible at one time and completely impossible another. One morning I had breakfast with Beth, who throughout our entire time together that morning appeared visibly skeptical about the ability to control diet with willpower alone. While I haven't described the method to her in great detail at the time, she made the following statement: "Subconscious belief systems that drive behavior and often conflict with our best intentions" will be in the way of your ability to successfully control your weight (and weight *loss*). Beth's attempts to lose weight were not as fruitful as some of the others I interviewed for this book. Although I couldn't tell, she was the heaviest she had ever been. Beth does not look overweight, but apparently she *feels* that way, and you could not argue with her. If she had asked me, I wouldn't suggest that she needed to lose weight, but she felt she did. Over the past 20 years she tried losing weight. At times she lost 10-15 pounds but shortly thereafter gained them back. Beth also told me of a long personal history of not feeling comfortable in her own body, suffering from food allergies, and constant stress, hence her inability to control her diet was contributed to other things going on in her life ("subconscious belief systems that drive behavior"), and hence her skeptical demeanor when I talked about controlling weight using your willpower.

Prof. Roy Baumeister of Florida State University explains this[33]. In a study conducted in his lab, he invited one group of students to eat cookies and another group of students to resist them and eat radishes instead. He then gave both groups an impossible puzzle to solve. Those who ate the cookies worked on the puzzle for 20 minutes on average before they gave up, while those who had to avoid the cookies (that were sitting right in front of them) and ate radishes instead gave up after only 8 minutes, on average. His conclusion was that willpower is a *limited resource*. The students that had to avoid cookies used a lot of that resource just to avoid the cookies. As a result, they didn't have enough willpower left to try at the puzzle longer. He further found that the same resource provides energy not only to exercise willpower but also to make *decisions*. So when you are in an environment in which you need to make many decisions, you will not have enough willpower left to control a successful diet. It is easier to avoid something to eat in the *morning*, when your willpower "container" is full, than it is after a long day full of decision-making and other willpower-depleting activities. You simply "don't have it in you" to avoid that treat. And at the worst time, what you eat in the evening will stay with you longer than what you eat in the morning.

Baumeister also made a discovery that would not help us much here. He found that glucose, responsible for carrying energy to the brain (and thus referred to as "fuel for the brain"), increases the

---

[33] http://www.apa.org/monitor/2012/01/self-control.aspx

amount of willpower (and self-control) you have. He claimed that people who exercised self-control tasks reduced their blood glucose level and, as a result, low glucose levels were a good predictor of poor self-control tasks, while eating and increasing the blood glucose level would increase your self-control abilities. This is problematic because eating less is exactly what we are trying to control here, and less food is exactly what reduces our ability to maintain the willpower to eat less—a predicament.

One takeaway from this research is that before attempting a diet that relies on your abundance of self-control, you need to ask yourself if you are at a point in your life in which you have other significant distractions that might deplete your reserves of *willpower*. If the answer is positive, then you need to see if you can change your life such that those distractions will go away, or simply decide that this is not the right time to embark on this diet. When I decided to start my Ph.D. program in 2004, I was the general manager of a $100 million business unit in Texas Instruments. It was a highly operational role and life was busy. I had to make decisions 24 hours a day. One morning, before school started, I woke up at 4am in cold sweat wondering if I was too crazy to take on Ph.D. studies at that time. By 7am I had completely withdrawn myself from the program. But in 2007, when I was the *strategist* for TI's wireless business unit, life was much easier. I had willpower to spare. I re-applied to the program, and three years later I received my Doctorate degree. There is the *right* time for everything, and there is the *wrong* time for everything, including a diet. If this is not the time in which you have enough willpower to start (the beginning is the hardest), try later.

However, the diet I described in this book has two provisions that can help. The first is the concept of "give the keys to someone else." I discussed several ways to do that, but essentially, to use Prof. Baumeister's terminology, this element reduces the requirements and use of willpower. In fact, this explains why "giving the keys to someone else" works. If the decision is not in *my* hands, I'm not really making it and, thus, am not depleting my willpower reservoir or requiring a certain amount of it to exist. The second is the premise of habit. The more your diet and exercise routines become habits, the less willpower is required to maintain them. They become easier. Imagine yourself trying to develop two hard habits at the same time. Wouldn't you fail in both? Try and develop one habit at a time.

9.

WHAT WORKED FOR ME MAY NOT WORK FOR YOU, BUT ...

When you are on board a cruise ship, you are a captive audience, which means they will try to sell you anything, anytime, all the time. I typically don't fall for that. However, as I was very involved with my diet at that time, I decided to take the class (free) about metabolism and toxins, as well as a toxin assessment (not so free). The instructor (who later gave me the toxin assessment) was a picture of good health and in top physical shape. From South Africa, he looked like someone who runs a marathon before breakfast and lifts trucks after lunch. This is what you wanted to look like. He explained the impact of toxins on metabolism and weight. He drew pictures and explained everything very clearly with drawings and a very exotic accent. Of course, the most important thing was for me to sign up to the $90 assessment of the level of toxins in my body using a Body Composition Analyzer[34].

---

[34] A few sources for the type of tests described here and how to interpret the results can be found in the following:
http://www.tanita.eu/uploads/media/1363267828_issuu.pdf
http://facstaff.bloomu.edu/jandreac/Downloads/class_notes/Exercise_You/Summer06/TANITA-Printout.pdf
http://www.unm.edu/~lkravitz/Article%20folder/underbodycomp.html
http://www.scalesgalore.com/printout.htm
http://ajcn.nutrition.org/content/33/1/27.full.pdf

Interested in my health recently, I signed up and showed up at my scheduled time. First, he explained that he would be measuring the amount of water in my body, or my Total Body Water (TBW) percentage. He explained that men have 50% to 65% water in their bodies while women have 45% to 60%. However, he prepared me, *my* test was not going to show less than 65%. Not even near it. The reason is that some of the water molecules are attached to the toxins and fat in my body and, thus, not measurable by his equipment. Based on that difference, we would be able to calculate the level of toxins in my body and able to determine a course of action. I couldn't wait for him to measure. I told him I was on a diet and that I had lost thirty pounds, but he quickly dismissed it and said that there are probably still toxins in my body and that the weight loss has likely done nothing to combat those. I felt discouraged. He then went on to explain the different remedies that are offered on the ship for a *special* price (more than $300 a month) that was only available during the cruise (of course! Especially when there was no Internet connection to verify that). He went on and on while I patiently waited for him to actually run the test.

Finally he placed the electrodes on me. He entered my age, my BMI (Body Mass Index: the ratio between height and weight), my weight, and other parameters and pressed a few final buttons. I heard a few beeps. Then the machine started printing something. He looked at the printout and didn't seem too happy with the results.

"What is the percentage of water?" I asked.

"65%."

"Isn't that what I'm supposed to have?"

"Yes."

"So, how much toxin do I have in my body?"

"None."

He was visibly disappointed. The entire conversation about the treatment and why a mere diet couldn't lower the amount of toxins had just become moot. My dieting worked.

***

Since my doctor suggested I write this book, it was only natural that I would ask him for the blood work results *before* and *after* that diet. Just to prove the effectiveness of this diet, I have included some of the results.

On July 3, 2012, days before I started this diet, my total cholesterol level was 189 mg/dL (it needs to be under 200 mg/dL, so it wasn't too bad), and on January 9, 2013, about a week after I reached my 200-pound goal, it was 165 mg/dL—better but not impressive. The ratio of LDL ("bad Cholesterol") to HDL ("good Cholesterol) has improved from 2.85 to 2.44. Better, but this too is still unimpressive. The best improvement was with my triglycerides level, which was at 177 mg/dL only days *before* the diet started (they need to be under 150 mg/dL) and at 86 mg/dL days *after* I reached my weight goal. That really impressed my doctor to the point that he took me off most of my medications and, specifically, my cholesterol controlling medications.

***

The preamble to this chapter shows that my weight loss program worked for *me*. It didn't cost me anything. I didn't buy books, DVDs, or fitness equipment that I didn't already have. I didn't get consultations other than my annual physical exam. And, I didn't make new memberships in a gym.

I mentioned at the beginning of this book that I assumed that you already know what you need to do to lose weight, and the issue is really one of *motivation*. Losing weight is hard, and it can't miraculously be made easy, so it needs to be matched with stronger and ongoing motivation to be successful. This is what this book is about—really.

However, once I did create the right *motivation* for myself, I had to implement things to help me lose weight. The rest of this chapter contains a list of all the things that worked for *me*. I cannot guarantee that they will work for you. *Your* body and your metabolism are different than mine. Some of the things below are "generally acceptable." Some might be less so. It is provided to you "as is" to try to help you to decide for yourself. Other things, not listed here, not tried by me, will probably work just as well, if not better. I don't claim to be an authority on how to lose weight. Only on how to get *motivated* to do so. This chapter is a hodge-podge of advice in different areas from nutrition to exercise. These are things that other people (mostly specialists) told me, and things I picked up myself through getting to know my body and metabolism better. There is no silver bullet. I bet that you already know a lot of those things and likely more things that I don't know, so feel free to skip reading this chapter and go right to the last chapter. Or, see if anything you find here may be useful.

∗∗∗

I was born and raised in Israel. My parents' generation was mostly a generation of immigrants, and most immigrants into Israel came from Europe. My parents were both born in Romania but met in Israel. My mother came on a ship that was seized in 1947 by the British Navy, and she spent a few months in a refugee camp in Cyprus until the United Nation's decision to create the state of Israel on November 29, 1947. At that time, she and her family were put on a ship and came to Israel, right in the middle of the Independence War. My father came to Israel in 1950. They both hung out in a group of other immigrants from Romania, and that's how they met. Immigrants typically bring cultural, traditional, and habitual elements from their original countries, and those would typically last for generations. Add to that the much shorter distance between Israel and Europe compared to the much longer distance between Israel and America, and it is easy to see why Israel diets and food preferences are influenced by Europe much more than the US. Things have changed since then: the dependency of Israel on the US since the oil and arms embargo of the 1970s and the beginning of the Foreign Military Funding that started after the Israel-Egypt peace accord in 1977 has grown Israel and the US closer. Airfare between the countries became more reasonable, and the boom of Israeli technology companies filing for IPOs (Initial Public Offerings) in the US stock exchanges in the 1990s only increased the cultural exchanges between the two countries. However, every now and then you still see signs that Israel is geographically closer to Europe than to the US. In early 2002, while we were visiting Israel (we lived in the Silicon Valley at that time), I considered a job offered to me in Israel. I met the Chief Operating Officer of a public technology company at a Starbucks. We sat for three hours as she was "selling" me on the company, the need for change, and the CEO. That was the only time I sat at a Starbucks in Israel. Starbucks opened its first location in Israel in August of 2001 and closed its last one in April of 2003—less than two years later. Israelis don't drink *American* coffee. They don't enjoy coffee the way Americans do. They enjoy coffee the way Europeans do.

And why am I telling you all of this? Because the Europeans eat a big *lunch*, and the Americans eat a big *dinner*. My belief is that you have 12-14 hours to burn what you ate at breakfast. You have 7-10 hours to burn what you ate at lunch, but you only have a couple of hours to burn what you ate at dinner. Remember, the title of this book is *The Worst Diet Ever*, so I don't need to conduct a clinical trial to show that my idea of a diet is better than anyone else. However, there is actual scientific support to my claim here.

There is a British adage that my British administrative assistant, Diana, keeps telling me: "Eat breakfast like a king, lunch like a prince, and dinner like a pauper." It does sound kind of British. Here in the US, it would probably sound like "Eat breakfast like a hedge fund manager, eat lunch like a Senator, and eat dinner like the other 99%." She didn't make it up. I don't know who did. But it is true, and there is logic behind it. In 2013, the results of a study conducted at Tel-Aviv University[35] were published in Obesity magazine[36]. The researchers compared weight loss from two diets of 1,400 calories each, one with the majority of calories consumed at *breakfast* and

---

[35] Jakubowicz, D., Barnea, M., Wainstein, J. and Froy, O. High Caloric intake at breakfast vs. dinner differentially influences weight loss of overweight and obese women. Obesity 2013 Mar 20. doi: 10.1002/oby.20460.
[36] http://doctorsonly.co.il/wp-content/uploads/2013/07/Jakubowicz-at-al-Obesity-2013-oby20460.pdf

Yoram Solomon

one with the majority of calories consumed at *dinner*. Overweight and obese women with metabolic syndrome were randomly assigned to one of the two weight loss groups: the *breakfast* group (700-calorie breakfast, 500-calorie lunch, and 200-calorie dinner) or the *dinner* group (200-calorie breakfast, 500-calorie lunch, and 700-calorie dinner). The diets were conducted over a period of 12 weeks. The high calorie breakfast resulted in greater weight loss and waist circumference reduction. Fasting glucose, insulin, and ghrelin (a hunger hormone) were overall reduced in both groups, but they were decreased to a significantly greater extent in the high calorie *breakfast* group. Average triglyceride levels decreased 33.6% in the breakfast group but increased by over 14% in the dinner group. Results from an oral glucose tolerance test and the overall daily glucose, insulin, ghrelin, and hunger scores were significantly better in the *breakfast* group. The breakfast group also reported a higher average satiety score than the dinner group. Based on the results of this study, a high-calorie breakfast with reduced intake at dinner may be beneficial for the management of obesity and metabolic syndrome in overweight and obese individuals.

Alex eats differently. Alex likes having dinner with his family. His daughters are young enough that he can still enjoy a family dinner. He eats light in the morning (apples and rice cakes), sometimes skips lunch (or gets only a snack), but eats a full dinner with his family. He probably can lose more weight (or maintain his weight) with less effort if he changed to a heavier breakfast and a lighter dinner, but that would probably not happen until his daughters stop having time for a family dinner anymore. Keep in mind that even the group in the Tel-Aviv University research that had a 700-calorie dinner lost weight because the participants in that group still maintained an overall 1,400-calorie daily limit. Alex counts and tracks his calorie intake every day.

And if you cannot avoid dinner, especially when it is part of a social event? For that instance there is the "morning after" remedy. This relies on the fact that your body will not be able to completely absorb your food and store it as fat over a single night. Some will still be available tomorrow. So, either try to work out as soon as you get back home (if possible, as this might be late at night and bother others at home) or work out early in the morning. Workout twice the day after, and eat less—much less. I had days in which I got home to find that I gained over five pounds that day (compared to the same measurement the night before), but given my metabolism, extra workout the following day, and much less to eat the following day, I could get rid of most or all of that extra weight before my body got used to it.

***

People gain ten to fifteen pounds on average during a cruise. Everybody knows that. If you've ever been on one, you know what I'm talking about. If you haven't, here is what to expect. Some of the restaurants are open 24 hours a day. You can get a hamburger, pizza, hot dog, ice cream, and more all day and all night. Then there's the breakfast buffet—actually, a dozen buffets in every food style you can imagine. There is almost nothing you can't get. Lunch is the same, only worse. There's more food at lunch. And then comes the almost-formal dinner: typically a three-course meal in a fancy restaurant with desert—or several. You simply eat all the time. You go to the pool and you eat. You go to see the show, have dinner before, and have a snack after.

                                    Yoram Solomon

Now, the ships have very nice fitness centers in them, but who goes to the fitness center when on a cruise? Isn't the whole idea of a cruise to have *fun* rather than to work out? Of course, you will see the triathlon and marathon runners working out but not you! Well, we went on a cruise on December 30th, 2012. I had met my goal the day before, and for the first time in many years my weight was less than 200 pounds. I was not going to gain ten to fifteen pounds that week. After all, I worked hard for it and, unlike my 1911 story, the plan was to keep the weight under 200 pounds for a long time. It was not enough just to get there. But it was going to be a challenge. And I was up for it. There was a lot to lose this time. If I had gained ten pounds during that cruise, it could take me a month or more to lose it again—a month in which I would not be able to buy, build, or fly my planes. The other challenge was that there was no scale I could use on the ship. So whatever I did, I had to give it my best and hope I was doing it well, but I also had to know that only after the cruise is over I would know what the results were.

So how do we do this? First of all, I decided to never go for *seconds.* I filled a reasonable size plate at breakfast and lunch. I first scouted all the buffet sections available without taking anything on my plate. Then, once I knew what was available, I filled one plate with my favorite food. I finished it, and that was it. No seconds. Same for lunch. Dinner was a bit trickier as it was *served.* Still, you can refuse things. The Royal Caribbean cruise we were on had a special *healthy* menu you could ask for, which offered meals with less than 600 calories (I don't know, maybe all cruises have it and I just never noticed it before). I chose everything from that menu. Half the time I skipped desserts. And they looked good. But there was too much at stake. I was not going to gain ten to fifteen pounds. No way.

There are plenty of activities onboard the ship, but I decided I will go to the gym three times a day. I went in the mid-morning. I went right after lunch, and I went right after dinner, and before the daily variety show. Maybe twice during that cruise I worked out less than three times a day. All other days I worked out three times. Every time I worked out, it was for some 30-35 minutes, and according to the treadmill, I burned 500 or more calories every time. So my daily workout had a total of 1,000 to 1,500 calories, and sometimes even more. Our room attendant was impressed with me, but I didn't do it to impress him. I did it so I can continue and buy, build, and fly my airplanes.

We drove back home from our arrival port of Galveston, Texas. As soon as we got home, I stepped on the scale. I lost a pound and a half during that cruise.

***

Do you ever feel stuffed right after a heavy meal? Do you then immediately wonder why did you have to eat so much? After all, it is not a comfortable feeling, and you want to lose weight anyway, so why eat too much, and what can you do about it?

You may have heard this advice before: eat *slowly*. Chew slowly. Try to stretch your meal for 20 or 30 minutes, and you will feel full with less food in your stomach. The rule, according to an article published in a 2010 issue of the Harvard Mental Health Letter[37], doesn't work all the time, but when it does, the article claims, it works because of the brain and not the digestive system. We *feel* full,

---

[37] http://www.health.harvard.edu/blog/why-eating-slowly-may-help-you-feel-full-faster-20101019605

                                        Yoram Solomon

or stuffed, or hungry, or simply satisfied due to signals transmitted to our brains from the gut through a nerve that connects them. However, it takes some time for the gut to start transmitting the message "I'm full" to the brain[38]. This message *will* be transmitted, eventually. If you eat slower, you give the food a chance to arrive at the gut, for the gut to transmit that signal to the brain, and for the brain to let you know that you are full and satisfied. If you eat too fast, you continue to send more food to the gut, and by the time the gut sends the message to the brain, there is more of food still going from your stomach to your gut—much more. And by the time that food arrives, the signal transmitted to the brain is no longer one of satisfaction, but rather one of "too much food."

Sometimes it might not be easy to eat slowly. Some foods can get spoiled if on the plate for too long or just not taste as good anymore (steak, for example). So you have to eat those quickly. What I do is decide upfront how much I should eat to feel satisfied. By now, I know my body well enough to make that determination. So I put that amount on my plate and eat it (even if I eat it fast). Then I stop, and for the next 20 minutes I tell myself "I *will* feel full. I will feel full. I will feel full." And then it happens. I feel full, not too full.

***

It is only fair, since this journey had begun at the TODAY show in NBC studios, that we visit there again. As I began writing this book, a piece on the TODAY show on April 22 caught my atten-

---

[38] http://www.livestrong.com/article/480254-how-long-does-it-take-your-brain-to-register-that-the-stomach-is-full/

tion[39]. Prof. Brian Wansink[40] of Cornell University and the former executive director of the USDA's Center for Nutrition Policy and Promotion talked about "tricking your mind" to feeling full after eating *less.*

In an experiment he conducted at the NBC studios he offered free food to the audience but in two different buffet settings. In one setting, he gave them normal size plates, normal size serving spoons, offered fruit and vegetables first, and fatty food (pasta) at the end. In the second setting, he gave them slightly *larger* plates, slightly larger serving spoons, and changed the order of food to offer the pasta *first* and the healthier fruits and vegetables at the end of the buffet table. Overall, the food was exactly the same. The second group consumed 56% more food and most of it was pasta. The first group consumed on average 890 calories while the second group consumed 1520 calories of pasta alone. Wansink claims that "we eat with our *eyes* and *minds,* not with our stomachs."

Wansink's work stands in contradiction to Sandra Aamodt's, who claimed that our brain will bring our weight back to a *predetermined* set point all the time. According to Wansink, we can trick our brains. It might be more short-term and address one meal at a time, but if you continue to implement the same short-term strategy over and over again, it becomes the norm and the long-term *habit.*

***

---

39 http://www.today.com/news/experts-say-you-can-trick-your-mind-helping-you-lose-2D12178338
40 For more about Brian Wansink's work go to:
http://www.mindlesseating.org/

                    Yoram Solomon

Combining Wansink's concept of "tricking your mind" with my concept of "give the keys to someone else," puts you in a situation where you will have limited access to food (although probably ample access to water). We have a vending machine at the office. So I make sure I rarely have bills or coins under $10. I hate to put $10 (or more) bills in a vending machine. I can ask someone for change, but I hate doing that as well. So this little *inconvenience* effectively puts the vending machine out of my reach. We held our planning meetings of the TEDxPlano event at Corner Wines[41], and I noticed that, although I had ample access to wine, my access to cheese and crackers (and chocolates, and truffles, and anything Jim had put on the table) depended upon *where* I sat near the table. When I sat at the head of the table, access was limited. Asking someone to pass the cheese was *inconvenient.* Even if only by a little, it meant that I had less cheese and, given that we held our meetings in the evening, lower consumption meant less weight gain. *Accessibility* to food can play a major role in how much you eat. Make food as inaccessible as possible when you don't really need it. Even adding little inconvenience can make a big difference.

***

One thing that I got from the nutritionist I met for six months after my Boston Heart Lab test was to look for cereals that have a carb-to-fiber ratio lower than 5 to 1. This means that you must choose food in which for every 1 gram of fiber there could be no more than 5 grams of carbohydrates, as listed on the nutritional value label. The Harvard Health Blog suggests an even lower re-

---

[41] Credits to my friends, Jim and Lynda McDevitt, owners of Corner Wines in Plano: http://www.cornerwines.com/

striction, with a ratio of 10 to 1 (for every 1 gram of fiber there could be no more than 10 grams of carbohydrates)[42]. I go with the more restricting ratio of 5 to 1. I have found quite a few whole grain foods that have a ratio better than that.

***

Exercising can be monotonous and boring. I see many people exercise with headphones, listening to music. However, we are talking about working out for the rest of your life. My entire playlist has just over 500 songs. As we grow older, new music might not appeal to us, so we are starting to play the same songs over and over again. This becomes monotonous and boring as well. My trick there is to have my iPad (remember that I work out at home, so I have Wi-Fi access) with headphones, and I watch YouTube videos, TED videos (especially since I was one of the organizers of the first TEDxPlano event), Netflix videos and movies, and any other videos of interest. There is always new video content created, and it can be engaging enough that I sometimes forget to increase (or even reduce) the speed and incline of my treadmill. Videos are, therefore, never monotonous and boring. And I get to learn new things—two birds with one stone.

***

The Israeli Defense Forces (IDF) always used the term "water discipline." Except that it meant different things at different times. Until about a year before my basic training at IDF, "water discipline" meant that soldiers had to endure long periods of time *with-*

---

[42] http://www.health.harvard.edu/blog/the-trick-to-recognizing-a-good-whole-grain-use-carb-to-fiber-ratio-of-10-to-1-201301145794

                              Yoram Solomon

out water. It was assumed that during war water might not be available all the time, and soldiers needed to be trained to live without it. That proved to be a bad idea as about a year before my basic training a soldier had died from dehydration. At that time, the meaning of "water discipline" had turned. It was now the need to drink a *large* amount of water whenever your sergeant told you to. And that happened quite often. Luckily, this overshoot didn't amount to cases of *water intoxication*, in which large amounts of water are absorbed by the body without any nutrients, which can cause death as well.

But during my basic training I got used to drinking large amounts of water. I now use this ability to lose weight. Drinking plenty of water makes your body feel full. Drinking at least two full glasses of water right before a meal would not cause water intoxication, but will prevent you from eating too much. Your gut and stomach will send the message "I'm full" to your brain earlier.

In 2003, a team of nine scientists measured the effect that water consumption has on metabolism[43]. They took a small group of participants, made sure they all fasted for 12 hours prior to the experiment, and that they didn't drink any water for 90 minutes before it started. Then they asked the participants to drink 500 ml of water and measured their energy expenditure (through measuring the amount of oxygen intake and carbohydrate output, among other things). Ten minutes after drinking water, energy expenditures started rising, and 60 minutes after drinking water it was 30% higher than before drinking it. With women, after 90 minutes the energy

---

43 Michael Boschmann, Jochen Steiniger, Uta Hille, Jens Tank, Frauke Adams, Arya M. Sharma, Susanne Klaus, Friedrich C. Luft, and Jens Jordan (2003) Water-Induced Thermogenesis:
http://press.endocrine.org/doi/pdf/10.1210/jc.2003-030780

expenditures went back to pre-water levels, while they were still slightly elevated with men a little while longer. Finally, even the water *temperature* seemed to have had an effect on energy expenditures: room-temperature water caused a much higher calorie burn than body-temperature water. The conclusion of the research was that drinking 1.5 liters of water a day would cause you to lose 200 calories a day due to faster metabolism more than without drinking that amount.

If we rely on the results of this research, the 30% impact would be the most effective during your workout routine. That's when you have the highest energy expenditure and when the 30% will, thus, help you lose the most. So, drink at least 500 ml of water about 30 minutes before you start exercising.

***

I really don't have a scientific support for what I'm about to say, but I found that my input versus output of liquids depends on what else I ate that day. The worst are pretzels and other sources of fine-grain processed wheat products. When I eat those, it's as if they *absorb* the water and turn into fat, as I have much less water coming out of me when I eat pretzels. For what it's worth…

***

Have you ever ordered a high calorie dish at a restaurant and a Diet Coke just to have someone make the sarcastic remark: "You are ordering a three thousand calorie dish and a Diet Coke?" Pointing out the absurdity of "saving calories" with your drink when you obviously didn't care much for the calorie intake of your meal? Well, a can of Coke has 140 calories in it. If you really ordered a 3,000-

Yoram Solomon

calorie meal, then the total would be 3,140 calories, which is more than 3,000 calories. So, yes, ordering a Diet Coke with a 3,000-calorie meal is still better than ordering it with regular Coke. When you find out how much effort is required on the treadmill (or any other type of workout) to lose those 140 calories (it takes me approximately 15 minutes, one mile at a speed of 4 miles per hour at an incline of 4%) you will appreciate the value of drinking a Diet Coke. I'm not suggesting that all your meals should have 3,000 calories, but regardless of the caloric content of your meals, every piece counts. So, I don't think it's hypocritical to order a 3,000-calorie meal with a Diet Coke. 3,000 calories are still less than 3,140.

***

It is sometimes harder to keep a routine when you travel. The easiest thing to do when you travel is to stop working out. After all, your convenient treadmill in your bedroom is not there with you. Working out in your underwear (just saying) is not appropriate, and you have a pretty busy day anyway. You didn't come here for pleasure; you came on business. Well, if you really want to, you can find the time to work out. Almost all hotels have fitness centers. So you have to wear shorts and a shirt. Big deal. There is room in your carry-on bag for that. And you will need to make the time in the day to do it. You'll be surprised how resourceful you can be when you fear the consequences of not meeting your daily/monthly goals (which are extrinsic, and someone else has the keys to them).

Meals while traveling are subject to the same rules as having to attend a dinner party. If you don't have a dinner meeting, avoid dinner as if you were home. If you do have a business or social dinner meeting, and you do not want to make the people at your table uncomfortable by not touching your food, either eat healthily (you will gain their respect by showing them that you have willpower) or eat normally and practice the "morning after diet" described above.

***

I think I have owned almost every type of pedometer that existed. This is probably because I like *technology*, and this piece of wearable technology looks really cool. At one point, I spent $149 to get the Nike Fuel Band bracelet. I wore it from the moment I got out of bed in the morning to the moment I got back in bed at night. It counted steps. It counted calories. It counted "fuel" (which I'm not sure how it related to anything). To some extent, it can meet most of the principles of my weight loss program: it provides me with extrinsic-external motivation. (There is an app that challenged me to reach certain goals. I would get virtual awards for having the highest workout day, best Thursday, best week, 25,000 points mark, and more. The motivation was to reach those goals.) The goals are daily and not long-term. You have the possibility to "give the keys to someone else" by posting your successes (or failures) on social media, and, thus, your friends keep you honest

However, the level of motivation is really weak compared with how hard it is to do the right things (eat less and exercise more), so it will not rise to change *habits*.

Maybe it shouldn't be a surprise that Nike announced closure of its Fuel Band group and discontinuation of the current and

Yoram Solomon

planned future product[44]. Those don't work for me. It doesn't mean they won't work for you.

***

When you go on the treadmill you ask yourself, how many calories do I need to burn so I will lose one pound? Common wisdom puts this number at 3,500[45]. If you burn 3,500 calories during your workout, you will lose one pound. For me, my 30 minute, 4.5 miles-per-hour, 6% incline, 2+ miles on the treadmill burns approximately 400 calories—or so the treadmill claims. This means that for me to lose one pound I will need to work out for over four hours. It could also mean that I can lose one pound a *week* this way, by working 30 minutes every day at the same level of intensity.

However, it is more complicated than that. There are interactions between your exercise, your eating habits, and your metabolism. And once again, *your* body is different than mine. Only once you start measuring your weight three times a day will you know what your exercise routine equates to in pounds lost. It is an interesting exercise to weigh yourself, then work out, and then weigh yourself again to see what was the effect of your workout routine on your body.

You also need to look at the workout routine as kick-starting the metabolism process for the day. If your workout is rigorous, your

---

44 http://www.cnet.com/news/nike-fires-fuelband-engineers-will-stop-making-wearable-hardware/

45 http://www.caloriesperhour.com/tutorial_pound.php and http://www.mayoclinic.org/healthy-living/weight-loss/in-depth/calories/art-20048065

body will continue to demand nutrition even after you completed your workout, and you will continue to burn calories.

Whenever I work out on the treadmill, I find that I lose weight at a rate of 1 pound for every 1,000 calories (not 3,500). There can be multiple reasons for that, one of which is that the treadmill, unaware of my weight and age, is giving me the wrong numbers. I still don't believe that it will give me one third of the number of calories I burned during one workout session. There could be interactions with other things, but it's still not 3,500 calories per pound. I found how effective workout is for *me*. You need to find out how effective workout is for *you*.

***

Friction can be very problematic for your exercise routine. I'm not talking about the mechanical friction in your training bicycle.

Product designers know that if there are too many steps required to get a product to work, or get it to do something you want it to, or too many clicks to get somewhere on a website, then people would not do it. Apple was very insightful in understanding the 80-20 rule (20 percent of functions are used 80 percent of the time) and eliminated the 80 percent of functions that will only be used 20 percent of the time, just so that access to those 20 percent will be so much easier. Less *friction*.

Exercise is the same. If it is *hard* to exercise, you won't do it. But we all have different preferences. Years ago, my wife and I bought an elliptical trainer. She heard that those are much better on the joints than treadmills. We used it briefly, and then it just collect-

Yoram Solomon

ed dust. I didn't like using it. I didn't like being the one dictating the speed and determining the resistance. So I didn't use it, and soon after neither did she.

I didn't work out for many years. At all. I would see my physician for annual checkups. Our conversation would go like this:

"Do you work out?"

"No."

"You know, you really need to work out."

"I do."

"So, why don't you work out?"

"I can never find the time." (Not true. I could find the time for much less important things, but I didn't *want* to. I neither like the elliptical nor the alternatives.)

"Will you start working out?"

"I'll try."

And we leave it at that. And I didn't work out. And a year later we would have exactly the same conversation. Deja vu.

After I left Texas Instruments in 2008 and joined Interphase, I decided to change. We already had a family membership at Lifetime Fitness for a couple of years, that would cost us close to 200 dollars a month, and we didn't do much with it. But this time it was different. I felt I wanted to start working out, so I chose swimming. I was a swimmer when I was in high school—serious swimmer—so I decided to use that as my workout.

However, there were logistics involved. I would need to think about everything I needed to take to the pool. I would drive to the facility, change, swim for 30 minutes or so, take a shower, and oops, I forgot to bring my underwear today. I need to go back home. And it was a pretty uncomfortable drive back home. Besides, the office was only a seven minute drive from my home, while the fitness center was fifteen. Just too much *friction.* Don's fitness facility was on his way to work. Less friction.

After only two months with the new company, in January of 2009, I stopped going to Lifetime Fitness every morning. I used to go during the weekend for one training session on the treadmill, but that was it. And that's not enough. But I did like the treadmill. It was maintaining the speed and incline for me, and all I had to do was to keep up with it. I liked it better than anything. Better than the pool. Better than exercise bikes. Better than ellipticals. *Much* better than ellipticals. We all have different preferences.

So in January of 2009 we went to Sears and bought a treadmill to put in our bedroom. And that was it. I probably worked out 80% of the time since then on that treadmill. I still do, more than five years later. I wonder when this treadmill will finally die. I work out almost every morning. Sometimes I work out in the evening instead. Sometimes both. My rate now is thirty minutes at a speed of 4.5 miles per hour and at an incline of 6 percent. This means I walk more than two miles every time and burn some 350 calories. Not too bad. But there is less *friction.* It is in my bedroom. I don't need to drive to it. I don't need to wait until it's available. I don't need to clean it. Heck, I don't even need to wear anything other than my underwear and running shoes. I must have walked more than 2,000 miles on that treadmill since we got it. I could have walked to Las Vegas and back, but it would have taken me six years.

It is all about eliminating *friction* from the process. I found that the best for *me* is a treadmill in my bedroom. This may not necessarily be what's best for you. Ask yourself what's the *least* inconvenient for you. After all, exercising is inconvenient by itself; let's at least not add things that will make it worse.

Your body and metabolism are different than mine. What works for me may not work for you, and vice versa.

Reduce friction from your daily workout, and add obstacles to your meals.

10.

IT'S YOUR TURN NOW

In the 175 days of my initial weight loss phase, from July 8 to December 29, there were only 12 days in which I was *above* the allowed weight limit. The worst was 1.7 pounds above the allowed weight limit. Only twice was I above the allowed weight limit for two consecutive days, but never more than two. On average I was 2.8 pounds *below* the committed weight level on every day. As you can imagine, towards the end of each month I had the lowest weight compared to the weight limit, as I was getting prepared for next month's weight limit and didn't want a disruption in my hobby. At best, I was 9.3 pounds under the weight limit, on July 31, as I initially worked really hard at it. Perhaps too hard.

***

I once spoke in a conference in Japan following Pat Gelsinger, the then Chief Technology Officer at Intel. I liked how he started his presentation. He said, "Let me first tell you what I'm going to tell you, then I'll tell you, then I'll tell you what I told you."

So let me now tell you what I told you. I will start by summarizing the assumptions and rationale for this approach to make sense:

- I assume that you already know *how* to lose weight through better nutrition and exercise, and if you don't, you know where and how to find out;

- If you learn what works for you and what doesn't, you will do *more* of the things that work and *less* of the things that don't;
- Intrinsic motivators (through the positive natural results of weight loss), albeit having high impact, are such long-term, that the Net Present Value of them is lower than the "cost" of the effort required to achieve those results;
- Single-milestone extrinsic motivation (using external "carrots and sticks" that have nothing to do with the benefits of weight loss) can be very effective, but just like climbing a hill, they will have a downhill side that will prevent long-term results;
- Measuring your weight several times every day will help you learn what works for you and what doesn't;
- Losing weight gradually over a long period of time can create new habits (unlike climbing a steep hill) that will be easier to maintain for the rest of your life.

In other words, the reason you weren't successful in losing weight until now (or was successful in losing weight but not in keeping that weight off for an extended period of time) was because you were looking for an *easy* diet that could be achieved with your very *weak* motivation (the low Net Present Value of your long-term health), and such an easy diet simply doesn't exist. The reason this diet will be successful is because it creates a stronger motivation to go through the hard effort required.

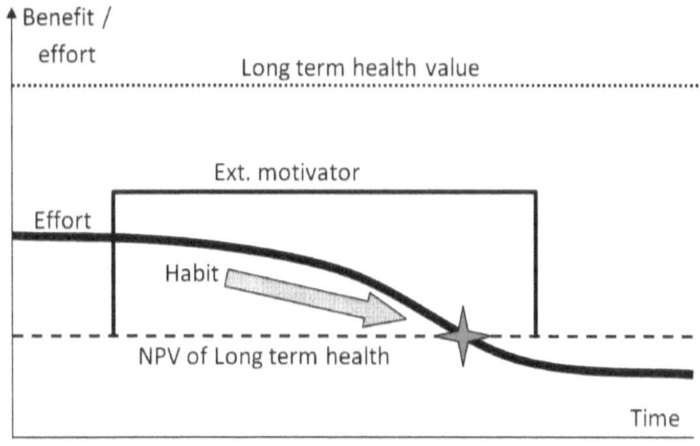

Figure 10: The worst diet ever

Let me repeat, one last time, the rationale behind the diet that worked for me and show what this process looks like over time. Figure 10 puts it all together. The benefit of long-term health has tremendous value to you. However, that value is discounted to today. The Net Present Value (NPV) of the long-term health is much lower today. It is vague and pales in comparison with the effort required to achieve it. That's why we cannot go through the weight loss effort without external "intervention." Once we add the *external* motivator (a motivator in the form of a reward that is contingent upon going through the weight loss effort, even though not a natural result of it), the combined benefit is higher than the cost of the effort. This will put the weight loss process in motion. Once this happens, and as long as it is a *daily* activity, consistently, the effort becomes *habit*. As it becomes habit, like every other effort (such as driving), it becomes *easier*. Then, at some point (marked in Figure 10 with a star), the *cost* of the effort, which by now became a highly engrained habit, becomes lower than the Net Present Value of your long-term health alone. At that point, and only at that point, you can eliminate the *external* motivation. Do it carefully, and add it back at the first sign that the habit gets reversed.

***

If, at some point, you feel that the effort is becoming smaller (as avoiding certain foods and working out are becoming *habits* and therefore easier), you can reduce the strength of the external motivator (replace external motivator I with external motivator II in Figure 11). You need to make sure that the *overall* motivation at that time (the new external motivator *and* the present value of your long-term health) is still higher than the effort.

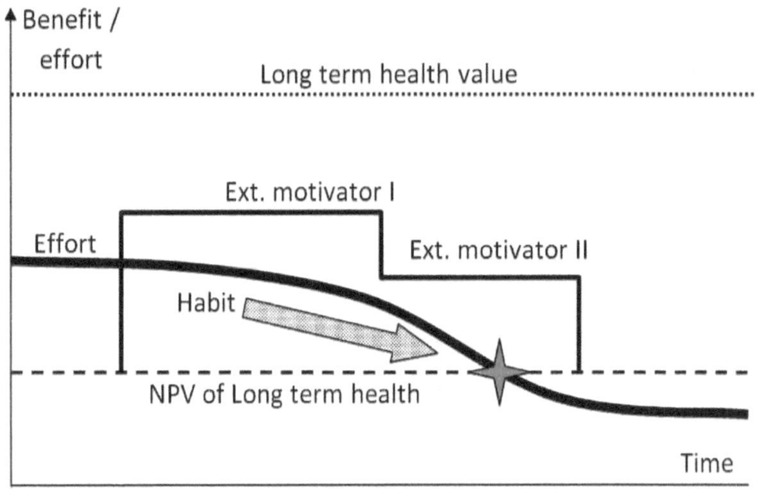

Figure 11: As the effort becomes a habit, the external motivator can be reduced.

One thing to watch out for, all the time, is whether the added external motivation is still *effective.* If you use your hobby, you might get tired of it. You need to make sure that the overall perceived benefit from the Net Present Value of your long-term health and the external motivator is still higher than the cost of the effort.

Yoram Solomon

When you feel your external motivator is not as effective (see Figure 12), replace that motivator with another external motivator that is more effective.

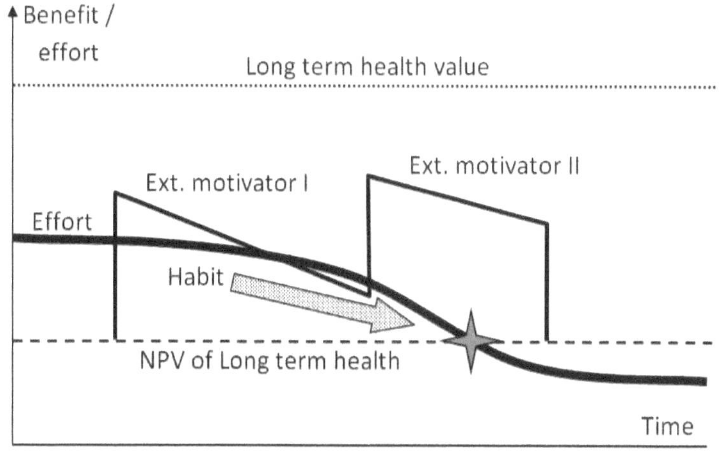

Figure 12: Sometimes the effectiveness of an external motivator declines, and it has to be replaced with a new motivator.

Finally, as you stay with your diet, and as you lose weight, you will start *feeling* better about yourself. You will *look* better. You will need fewer medications. You will feel more energy throughout the day. It will be easier to tie your shoelaces. Those things actually have a positive effect even on the perceived value of your long-term health (Figure 13). The better you feel now, the more you have to lose if you let yourself fall back to old eating and no-exercising habits. If you have more to lose, and if you like yourself better now, the intrinsic motivation from the Net Present Value of your long-term health (which is naturally linked to the weight loss effort) increases to the point you need less of an external motivation or need it for a shorter period of time.

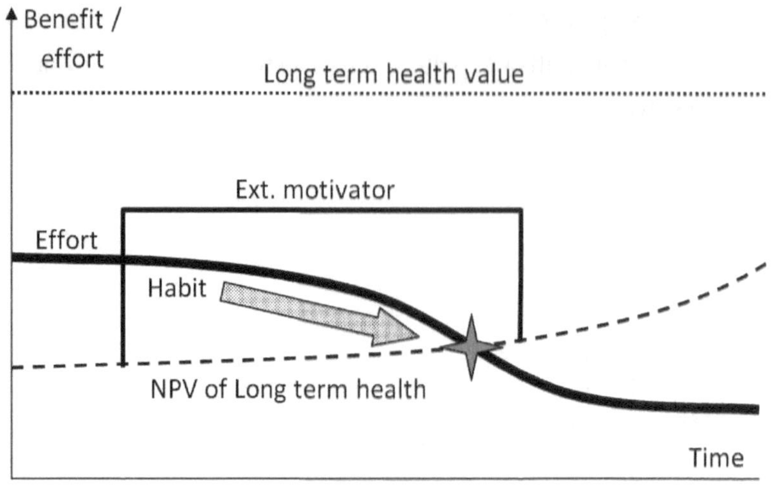

Figure 13: The effect of positive results on the present value of the long-term health

***

If the above makes sense, then there are five steps for this diet (five principles):

- First, set the *goal* and break it into 6 month steps. You don't want to achieve it too fast; you want to create new *habits* that will last for the rest of your life. You should have a "weight limit" for every month. Build your new routines (what you eat and when and how to exercise) into your most routine time of the day (typically the morning), with *cues* that exist every day at that time (such as the alarm clock in the morning for exercise).

- Second, weigh yourself at least three times a day. The first time in the morning will be the one that counts (and determine whether you are below the "weight limit" or not). The

Yoram Solomon

second time is as soon as you get home in the evening, when there is still a chance to do something about it. The third one: right before you go to sleep, to get a sense of what will you weigh in the morning. Through those frequent weightings, you will get to know *your* body and metabolism, how different foods affect you, and how exercise works out for you

- Third, you need to find an effective *extrinsic* motivator that, while not naturally and logically linked to the outcome of your weight loss efforts, will create *rewards* and *consequences* for meeting (or not meeting) the daily/monthly weight limits. Those rewards and consequences have to:
  - Be *significant* to you. They cannot be something that you don't really care about.
  - Affect you *every day*. Not in a way that will affect your earning potential, family life, or anything like that, but things that you enjoy.

- Fourth, give the keys to someone else. You cannot be trusted. You will cut corners and take shortcuts and, after all, the link between those rewards or consequences and weight loss is artificial. Give the keys (figuratively or literally) to someone who will not give them to you unless you meet your goals and will be really mean about it. This has to be someone you trust and respect and someone you will really feel very uncomfortable letting down.

● Fifth, when the consequences don't matter anymore, change consequences. It's OK to go for a period of time without consequences, as long as your new, healthy *habits* are in control, but as soon as you start slipping back to old habits, immediately apply a correction plan with new consequences.

Note one thing: I am not telling you what to eat and what not to eat. I'm not telling you how (or how much) to exercise. You will figure those out for yourself. There are plenty of diet and exercise regimens that will work for you. I wasn't trying to give you that *knowledge*. You already have it, and if you don't, you'll know where to find it. You're not stupid. The only thing you needed was the right *motivation*, and if you follow the advice in this book, I think you got it! Maybe, just maybe, this is not the *worst* diet ever. Good luck.

11.

WHAT EMPLOYERS, INSURANCE COMPANIES, AND GOVERNMENTS CAN DO

In the first ten chapters of this book I explained why the motivation to lose weight and live healthy must be *extrinsic.* Intrinsic motivation simply doesn't work here. The assumption in those first ten chapters, though, is that *you* are the one who wants to lose weight and live healthy. You still don't have enough intrinsic motivation to do it, so you needed extrinsic motivation, but it was still something that *you* wanted to do. I taught you how to motivate yourself.

However, the need for you to lose weight may not even be coming from you. You see, there are consequences of your lifestyle to others. Specifically, to the company you work in, to the insurance company that covers your healthcare, and to the economy of the country you live in. Those are incentivized as well to keep you healthy, sometimes even more than you.

It is estimated that the healthcare costs of obesity and the preventable chronic diseases that result from it are between $147 billion to $210 billion per year in the US alone. Obesity and its consequences cause absenteeism (estimated at $4.3 billion annually), and lower productivity, costing employers $506 per obese worker per year[46]. Furthermore, the healthcare costs for severely obese adults (BMI >40) are 81% higher than for healthy-weight adults. Emergency Room costs for severely obese patients are 41% higher than those for the healthy-weight patients. They are 28% higher for moderately obese patients, and 22% higher for overweight (albeit not obese) patients.

One report claimed that the medical expenditures and lost productivity as results of obesity could amount to $6,087 annually for men, and $6,694 for women. It further stated that individuals with BMI >35 represent only 37% of the population, but 61% of the excess costs[47].

Finally, a 2008 report showed that an investment of $1 in disease prevention would yield a return (in healthcare costs and productivity losses) of $5.60 on average in the US, with different states showing returns from $4.20 (Arizona) to $9.90 (Washington DC)[48].

One thing is clear—companies, insurance companies, and even governments are highly motivated to assure their constituents are healthy. Put aside the social and non-financial reasons—the financial motivation alone is enough.

Not all countries are affected by obesity in a similar way. According to a 2017 report by the Organisation[49] for Economic Co-operation and Development (OECD) the US leads the world signifi-

---

[46] https://stateofobesity.org/healthcare-costs-obesity/

[47] https://www.ncbi.nlm.nih.gov/m/pubmed/20881629/

[48] http://healthyamericans.org/reports/prevention08/

[49] Not a spelling mistake... It's a European organization.

     Yoram Solomon

cantly with 38.2% obesity rates among adults. The second closest country is Mexico, with 32.4%. The average among OECD countries is 19.5%, and the countries with the least obesity problems are Japan (3.7%) and Korea (5.3%)[50]. Of all the things we could lead the world in… But there is a reason. A study conducted by the Food Industry Center at the University of Minnesota credited the dramatically lower obesity rates in Japan (compared to the US) to the higher cost of food (causing Japanese people to consume 200+ less calories per day), and the higher cost of driving (causing them to walk more)[51]. The report makes the following recommendation:

> "In terms of policy solutions, economic incentives could be structured to encourage Americans to drive less and use public transportation more, which would typically also mean walking more."

In fact, this report makes a strong case for the point I'm about to make: entities (company, insurance company, and even government) can create extrinsic motivation to lose weight and live healthy. How can they do that?

***

Before I talk about the *How*, let me start with the *What*. As the beginning of chapter 5 clearly indicated—you must start with what you *measure*. Peter Drucker, the business guru, said: "if you can't measure it, you can't manage it." It's great to create a system of extrinsic motivation, but it has to be tied to a measureable outcome, and with targets. It could be weight; it could be the Body Mass Index (BMI) as described in the introduction; or any other measure of

---

[50] http://www.oecd.org/els/health-systems/Obesity-Update-2017.pdf
[51] http://ageconsearch.umn.edu/bitstream/14321/1/tr06-02s.pdf

health. For now, I would use BMI as the metric for health. WebMD[52] suggests that underweight people have a BMI <18.5. A healthy weight produces a BMI between 18.5 and 24.9. Overweight comes with a BMI between 25 and 29.9, while Obese is defined as a BMI of 30 or higher. Another distinction is that severely or morbidly obese people have a BMI higher than 40.

Using BMI is better than using weight (in my opinion, although I'm no health or diet expert—I'm only a motivation expert), because BMI takes other things into consideration. Having a 5' tall person and a 6'6" tall person target the same weight doesn't make sense. Also, asking a 300-lb person and a 150-lb person both to lose 100 lb. doesn't make sense either. Reaching the healthy BMI for their specific weight and height makes more sense to me. I would also think that involving more research and true medical opinion, whether in general or individually for every person would be desirable.

But for the following discussion, I will use BMI as the metric, and the healthy BMI range (18.5 – 24.9) as the target.

***

What can a company do?

As one of the reports cited above claimed, obesity costs more than $6,000 per person annually in healthcare expenses and productivity losses. Further research is needed, but hypothetically I will assume that the true loss to the company is only $4,000 of the $6,000. It is manifested as revenue decline, increased costs, and increase in

---

[52] http://www.webmd.com/men/weight-loss-bmi

the healthcare insurance premiums that the employer pays, and possibly other costs.

How much should the company be willing to spend to compensate for that cost? In this day and age of Corporate Social Responsibility (CSR), I could claim that companies would be willing to spend *more* than $4,000, due to the non-financial social value of healthy employees. Another possibility would be to assume that companies would be willing to do no more than break even, which means they would be willing to spend $4,000 to eliminate the $4,000 loss, while keeping their employees healthy.

However, I will go further and take the Milton Friedman approach that the purpose of a business is to maximize profits to shareholders. If the company spends nothing to extrinsically motivate its employees to be healthy, it would lose $4,000 due to the costs of obesity. If it spends $4,000—it will lose those $4,000 (albeit the employees will be healthy). I will claim to you that the incentive required to lose weight and live healthy is worth less than $4,000 annually. I base that on the Bureau of Labor statistic that the average US salary is $44,148 annually for a 40-hour work week. The average management salary is $63,076, and the average service salary is $28,080[53]. The $6,000+ cost of obesity mentioned above is the US average, and therefore it represents 14.5% of the average salary. And here comes the 200 billion dollar question—would 14.5% increase to your salary be enough extrinsic motivation to complement the net present value of your intrinsic motivation and get you to lose weight? Would it amount to the black bar in Figure 4? I believe the

----

[53] https://www.thebalance.com/average-salary-information-for-us-workers-2060808

answer is definitely *yes*. But I also believe that the answer would still be yes if the bonus amount was only 5% of your salary. The economics work. Companies could save $4,000 of losses resulting from unhealthy employees, by paying them only $2,000 to be healthy. The fact that they would have healthy employees is just the icing on the cake. OK, maybe not cake. Maybe a salad. And maybe not icing, but rather low-fat dressing…

There is another method that comes to mind, maybe even more effective. You are familiar with the Biblical "God has given and, therefore, God can take away." In comes the Broaden-and-build theory[54] which, in a nutshell, states that the effect of a negative event is three times more powerful than the effect of a positive event. As a result, what if the paycheck includes a 5% "health premium" that would be taken away if an employee cannot maintain a healthy BMI? Taking the 5% away is three times more powerful than giving those 5%. In fact, if I'm right and giving 5% bonus is enough, then maybe taking 1.67% of a salary (pre-designated as "health premium" so it can be taken away without leading to litigation…) for "unhealthy behavior" would be as impactful as giving 5% for "healthy behavior?" I haven't done the research, but I suspect it is worth doing.

If the metric is BMI, it is important that the extrinsic motivator will be tied well to the target, healthy BMI. Employees should not be compared against each other for their BMI performance. An idea I heard was to give bonuses (or not remove the "health premium" salary element) only to the top 20% of employees who meet their BMI targets. This might cause unhealthy behavior such as bulimia.

---

[54] https://positivepsychologyprogram.com/broaden-build-theory/

I would recommend having a gradual scale of bonuses (or removal of such). If my BMI is 40 now, my target is below 25, and my positive bonus (or lack of negative deduction) kicks in only once I reach 25—I might just give up, considering it a mountain too high to climb. However, if I get 50% of my bonus as long as I'm below BMI of 35, and 100% below 25, I may be incentivized all the way. 50% is better than nothing, and 5 BMI points (30 lb. for a 250-lb person) is much more achievable than 15 BMI points (95 lb. for a 250-lb person). The achievement of the intermediate goal (or goals) can provide additional motivation to reach the ultimate goal.

The metric can be dynamic, as well. Much like my own weight loss, in which I expected to be under a different weight every month until I reached my final target weight, companies can implement a sliding BMI scale. You may not want employees to lose more than 2 (for example) BMI points in a month, until they reached their target BMI, under 25. Remember that you also want to form new habits, and those are formed only over time. The amount of bonus given (or "health premium" not taken away) could be tied to the sliding monthly target, rather than the final target. This way, if my BMI at the beginning of this process was 39 (and my target is 25), I would be expected to have a BMI of 37 after the first month (and thus 100% benefit would be tied to a BMI of 37 that month), 35 in the following month, etc. This way, a BMI of 36 in the first month would entitle me to 100% of the benefit, but the following month the same BMI would only entitle me to 50% of the benefit. Until I reach my target BMI of 25. From that moment on, 100% of the benefit would only be given as long as the BMI is at or below 25.

A consideration could be whether to "punish" employees for going below a BMI of 18.5, which is considered underweight. I will leave this debate open. I personally believe that if there is no additional extrinsic motivation to go below 25, people would stop there. Maybe a little more so they don't accidentally lose their benefit over one party… But they will not be motivated (extrinsically or intrinsically) to go significantly below that.

As a final note on company incentives—those could be non-financial as well. I wouldn't recommend promotions as an extrinsic motivation to live healthy, as promotions should be job-merit related. However, other gifts and benefits could have a more significant value to employees than the financial cost to the company. I'm not sure what the value of a reserved parking spot is closer to the building entrance, but I can tell you with certainty that it's not zero. At the same time I can tell you that it doesn't cost the company anything to reassign parking spots. You get the idea.

***

Until now this chapter discussed how *companies* can create extrinsic motivation for employees to reduce the direct and indirect costs of obesity (productivity loss and employer-side health benefit costs). Now it's time to discuss two other interested entities.

The first is *healthcare insurance companies.* If premiums are fixed, then obese customers create higher costs to insurance companies. What if insurance companies could change your premiums based on your BMI (fixed or on a sliding scale)? Much like term life insurance premiums depend on your age and consumption of tobacco and alcohol? If it costs the insurance company $6,000 a year more if you are obese, wouldn't they be happy reducing your premium (or, better yet, your deductible) by $3,000? Wouldn't you mind if your premiums were $250 a month lower? Once again, a possibly more effective way would be to remove a benefit (such as a discount) if you don't meet the BMI goal rather than give you a benefit (such as a discount) if you don't. Three times more effective.

***

Finally, governments have their own motivation to increase public health. From the amount of subsidies they provide for healthcare benefits to reduced taxes due to lower productivity, and more. You also must remember that governments are employers, too, which makes whatever was relevant to companies above relevant to governments, as well.

The extrinsic motivation tools governments have may include changing tax brackets, special deductions (imagine getting a higher deduction the better your health or BMI are), and even refund schedules. Wouldn't you be (extrinsically) motivated enough to lose weight and live healthier if you could lower your taxes?

And before you yell that the government should not interfere with my health, let me remind you that *my* taxes are not the only source of revenue that pays for my poor health and the consequences from it. *Yours* do to. You would pay more taxes because I'm not willing to watch my health. Now, do you want the government to incentivize me to watch my health, if the results will eventually be lower taxes for you too?

***

Let me save you some time now. I'm sure you are about to start searching for laws and regulations that would prevent employers, insurance companies, and governments from interfering in our health, or tying parts of our salary, insurance premiums, or taxes on them. Don't bother. It's irrelevant. Even if such laws exist—they should be changed. My focus in this book and this chapter is not to identify what is *allowed,* but rather what could be *effective.*

***

The final questions are practical and logistical. How do you measure the health (or even more specifically weight or BMI) of your employees, customers, or citizens? Do you rely on self-reporting? Do they have to do it in front of a human resources manager, an insurance agent, or a government administrator? How often would you measure it?

There are answers to all those questions. The answers could vary from technological to psychological, and would change over time. I will leave it to you to determine the answers, as I leave you with the concept.

Yoram Solomon

APPENDIX: SURVEY SUMMARY

One day, as I was going through advanced course work in my doctoral studies, I received a call from my academic advisor.

"Do you need help with registration?"

"No, I'm fine. I already registered for the next quarter."

"I saw that. You know, by now you should probably already have a topic for your dissertation."

"Oh, I do. I have selected a topic."

"Well, then you should also discuss a *methodology* for your research with your mentor."

I should pause and explain here that there are two major research methodologies: *quantitative* and *qualitative*, with strong believers in each, that would completely discount any research done with the other. Quantitative research is *explanatory* in nature; based on developing (or using existing) surveys, conducting them on a large number of participants, and then performing statistical analysis on the results to support (or reject) hypotheses made. Qualitative research, on the other hand, is more *exploratory* in nature, and is based on a smaller number of face-to-face (mostly) interactive interviews, in which new information can be generated that may not have existed using a pre-determined set of survey questions.

"I already know what methodology I'm going to use."

At this point, he seemed annoyed with me and said:

"OK, let me be blunt, you registered for *both* quantitative *and* qualitative research classes, so you really don't know what you want to do!"

"But I do!" I replied: "I'm going to use qualitative, case study method."

"So why are you taking quantitative research classes as well?"

"It's simple. I will complete my dissertation using *qualitative* case study method. Then I get my Ph.D. Then, what will happen if at some point in life I will want to perform a *quantitative,* survey-based study? I will then realize that I never took quantitative research methods class?"

He claimed that nobody had done that before and checked with the head of the research department at the university, who didn't see anything wrong with what I wanted to do. So I took all research classes, quantitative *and* qualitative, including survey development, and went on to do a mostly qualitative dissertation (although it did have a few quantitative elements to it). Taking survey development and quantitative research classes will later prove important for the research included in this book.

✳✳✳

As I described earlier, I conducted the survey for this book between April 15 and April 23, 2014. My goal was to have 200 participants, constituting a good enough sample. I distributed the survey

Yoram Solomon

through my Facebook, LinkedIn, and Google+ networks. Within 8 days I had 222 responses to the survey and I closed it to begin analyzing it.

There were 10 questions in the survey.

1. Have you in the past five years (or today) wanted, needed, or were told that you need to lose weight?
- No
- Yes

The purpose of question 1 was to measure the awareness of the participants to losing weight and their perception of their own need to do so.

2. Have you in the past five years lost weight intentionally through diet and/or exercise? (Do not include weight-loss surgery in your answers)
- No
- Yes

Question 2 was created to filter the participants who did *not* lose weight from those who did, when applicable.

3. If you have lost weight—what is the closest to your total weight loss?
- Didn't lose weight, or less than 10 lb.
- 10 lb.
- 20 lb.
- 30 lb.
- 50 lb.
- 100 lb. or more

The third question measured the *dependent* variable (result, or outcome): how much weight was lost as a result of the effort. It should be noted that not all participants thought they *should* have lost a high value, and this question would have potentially be better off being replaced with *two* questions: how much weight did you *want* to lose, and how much weight did you *actually* lose, and then the ratio between them could have been used to measure how they met their goals.

4. If you lost weight—over what period of time did you lose it? (Choose the option closest to the time it took you to lose)
- Didn't lose weight
- 1 month
- 2 months
- 3 months
- 6 months
- 12 months or more

Question 4 measured an independent factor, to later correlate the ability of participants to keep their weight off to how fast they lost their weight. My hypothesis was that the participants who lost their weight too fast would have hard time keeping it off.

5. What motivated you to lose weight?
- I didn't lose weight
- My long-term health and/or well being
- An immediate health risk or life threat that needed to be taken care of now
- I promised myself that if I reach a milestone weight, I will award myself with something (example: buy a new car)
- I created a benefit for myself as long as my weight is under a certain value

The fifth question measured a second independent variable, a *categorical* one, to compare the different potential motivators on weight loss, as well as on the ability to keep the weight off.

6. Did you gain that weight (or part of it) back after a period of time?

- I didn't lose weight to start with
- I kept all the weight that I lost off
- I kept more than half of the weight I lost off
- I gained the weight I lost back
- I gained more than the weight I lost

Question 6 was a dependent variable (an outcome or result) to measure the sustainability of the weight loss effort over a long period of time.

7. How long has it been since you lost weight?

- For the last time—I didn't lose weight!!!
- LESS than 3 months
- MORE than 3 months but LESS than 6 months
- MORE than 6 months but LESS than a year
- MORE than a year

The purpose of question 7 was to sort participants into a group in which enough time has passed since the weight loss so that the answers to the question (6) whether they kept their weight off will be relevant.

8. How much money do you estimate you spent on weight loss products and services in the past five years? (You don't need to be exact. Weight loss products and services include books, pills/products, fitness equipment if this is the purpose you purchased

it for, memberships such as Weight Watchers or others, dietitian appointments, etc.)

- NONE, or LESS than $10
- MORE than $10 but LESS than $100
- MORE than $100 but less than $1,000
- MORE than $1,000

Both questions 8 and 9 were borne simply out of curiosity, to find out how much the participants spend on weight loss products and services (to potentially qualify the $200 national average described in the introduction), and to get a sense of the size of the market for this book.

9. Did you buy any weight-less related BOOKS in the past five years?

- No
- Only one
- More than one

10. Whether you lost weight or not, how often do you weigh yourself?

- Never, or Less than once a month
- Typically once a week
- Typically once a day
- More than once a day

Finally, question 10 measured the third independent variable, the *frequency* of weighing, and would be used to analyze the effect this frequency has on weight loss and the ability to keep the weight off for an extended period of time.

ACKNOWLEDGEMENTS

Although this book poured out of me, it was the help of other people who made it happen. I couldn't have done it without all the help I received.

First, I would like to thank the 222 anonymous survey participants who took the time to answer my survey questions. I don't know who all of you are, and you shall remain anonymous. I also thank you for your willingness to forward the survey to others and helping me reach (and exceed) my 200 participant goal so fast.

I would also like to thank Joe, Alex, Valerie, Beth, Don, and Matthew who shared their personal stories with me and helped refine, adjust, and clarify my theories. I truly appreciate your openness and your willingness to share your stories with my readers.

This second edition came out of a discussion I had with a new friend, Hidetaka Kai (Tak) from ConfluCore Japan. He was intrigued by the first edition of the book, and told me that in Japan companies (and even the government) would like to assure cost reductions associated with poor health. The discussion we held led to the newest chapter in this book, chapter 11. I thank Tak for that.

Maya, my smart and thoughtful now-college daughter, took the time to tally the survey responses, to tabulate them, and to give me the results that supported my hypotheses throughout this book, and even created new insights.

Shira, my down-to-earth practical then-middle-school daughter, offered me rare one-day coupons when I needed a break from meeting my goals but enforced their use very strictly.

I want to thank my personal physician, Dr. Sander Gothard of Village Health Partners in Plano, who followed my weight loss with advice, guidance, and shared with me the medical results of it. You keep me alive!

When writing this book, I was inspired by the work, research, theories, and provoking thoughts of Dan Ariely, Teresa Amabile, Karl Duncker, Sam Glucksberg, Charles Duhigg, Sandra Aamodt, Brian Wansink, Daniel Kahneman, and Amos Tversky. I owe each one of them a debt of gratitude for helping me understand things that would otherwise not make sense.

Finally, I want to thank *you*, my readers, for buying this book, reading it and, hopefully, taking a chance and using it to reach your health goals in a different way. Good luck!

ABOUT THE AUTHOR

Yoram Solomon received his Ph.D. in Organization and Management from Capella University in 2010. He spent two years researching why people are more creative in startup companies than they are in mature and large corporations. He used his insights to help companies and non-profit organizations create environments conducive to creativity. He is a multi-disciplinary professional, who also holds an electrical engineering associate degree, a law degree from Tel-Aviv University, and a Master in Business Administration from the University of Colorado in Colorado Springs.

Throughout his career, Dr. Solomon was mostly a strategist, an innovator, and an entrepreneur. He worked in a wide range of companies, from large Fortune 500 corporations (such as Texas Instruments) to small startup companies that he founded.

In 2015, Yoram was elected to the Plano Independent School District board of trustees. He is a graduate of Leadership Plano Class 31, a former board member in Plano Youth Leadership, and an Aerospace Education Officer (and former Pilot) in the Civil Air Patrol (US Air Force Auxiliary unit).

Born in Israel, served fifteen years in the IDF, moved to Silicon Valley for five years, where he joined a small company and sold it before he became a Vice President in PCTEL, a Senior Director of Strategy and Industry Relations in Texas Instruments, and then a

Vice President of Strategy at Interphase Corporation in Carrollton, Texas, where in 2010 he invented *penveu*, an innovative interactive display system developed for schools, and brought it to the market in 2014. Yoram and his wife and two daughters, Maya and Shira moved to Plano, Texas in 2003, and made it their permanent home, where he also became a member (and a board member) at the Plano Rotary Club, that puts service above self.

He is an avid article writer, and in 2007 published his first book: "Bowling with a Crystal Ball: How to Predict Technology Trends, Create Disruptive Implementations and Navigate them Through Industry," which became a textbook for a technology and industry forecasting class he developed and taught in the Graduate School of Management at the University of Texas at Dallas.

Dr. Solomon's passion for entrepreneurship put him on the board of the North Texas Alliance for Higher Education and Regional Center for Innovation and Commercialization, and he is a founding member of the North Texas Angel (investor) Network.

Yoram can often be found speaking passionately on variety of topics, including as a keynote speaker at Startup Weekend, and many other venues. In 2016 he became a professional member of the National Speakers Association at both the local level and the national level.

It is his strategic approach to everything that led to the weight loss program described in this book, which he proved on himself.

                                              Yoram Solomon

www.ingramcontent.com/pod-product-compliance
Lightning Source LLC
Chambersburg PA
CBHW031114250726
48655CB00004B/1702